Sirtfood Diet

The Ultimate Guide to Burn Fat, Lose Weight, Get Lean with 101 Carnivore, Vegetarian & Vegan Recipes. Discover the Secrets of Celebrities to Activate Your Skinny Gene & Feel Great

Adele Hamilton

TABLE OF CONTENTS

INTRODUCTION

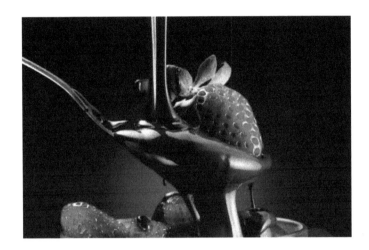

The sirtfood diet relies upon the possibility that particular nourishments impel sirtuins in your body, which are specific proteins speculated to receive various rewards, from protecting cells in your body from exacerbation to switching maturing. Nourishments allowed on the diet consolidate green tea, dim chocolate, apples, natural citrus products, blueberries, red wine, parsley, turmeric, kale, and tricks.

On the official Sirt food diet site, protectors explain that the diet has two "basic" stages. Stage one is seven days with daily involving three sort food green juices and one dinner stacked up with sirtfoods — a sum of 1,000 calories. You might be, to some degree, less starving on days four through seven when you're allowed to increase your admission to 1,500 calories with two dinners and two green juices.

Stage two isn't more reassuring. This stage continues for about two weeks, in which you are permitted to have three "balanced" sirtfood-rich suppers daily despite your one phenomenal green juice. The goal during this time is to progress further weight decrease. While the upsides of sirtuins seem to be empowered by all accounts, the sirtfood diet is promoted up till now, another way to deal with "shed seven pounds in seven days!" And you know now, that outrageous weight control doesn't work that way.

What appears as though a goody lifted directly from a science fiction movie, a 'sirtfood' is nourishment high in sirtuin activators? Sirtuins are a kind of protein that shields the cells in our bodies from failing miserably or getting aggravated through disorder. However, the study has shown they can help deal with your digestion, increase muscle, and consume fat.

The Sirtfood Diet book was first launches in the U.K in 2017. However, the U.S. arrival of the book brought about a greater interest in the diet. The diet began getting exposure when Adele appeared her slimmer figure at the Billboard Music Awards last May. Her mentor, Pete Geracimo, is a massive fan of the diet and says the vocalist shed 30 pounds from following a Sirt food diet.

What is Sirtfood?

Sirtfoods are recently found group of nutrient-rich foods which appear to be able to 'actuate' the body's skinny genes (otherwise called sirtuins), similarly as fasting diets do, with a similar scope of advantages, however without the regular drawbacks of fasting diets, for example, irritability, hunger, and muscle loss.

By eating a diet rich in Sirtfoods, it is asserted that participants will get thinner, gain muscle, look and feel good and possibly live a longer and increasingly healthy life.

What is SirtFood Diet?

The Sirtfood Diet is the better approach to move weight rapidly without radical dieting by initiating the same 'skinny gene' pathways generally just induced by fasting and exercise. Certain foods contain synthetic compounds called polyphenols that put mild stress on our phones, turning on genes that copy the impacts of exercise and fasting. Foods rich in polyphenols-including dark chocolate, kale, and red wine-trigger the sirtuin pathways that effect digestion, mood and aging. A diet rich in these sirtfoods launches weight reduction without sacrificing muscle while maintaining ideal health.

Add healthy sirtfoods to your diet for successful and sustained weight reduction, incredible vitality and sparkling health. Switch on your body's fat-burning powers, supercharge weight reduction and help stave off disease with this simple-to-follow diet created by the specialists in nutritional prescription who proved the effect of Sirt foods. Dark chocolate, kale, coffee - these are foods that actuate sirtuins and switch on the alleged 'skinny gene' pathways in the body. The Sirtfood Diet gives you a straightforward, healthy way for eating for weight reduction, delicious simple-to-make plans and an maintain plan for delayed success. The Sirtfood Diet is a diet of incorporation not avoidance, and sirtfoods are widely affordable and available. This is a diet that urges you to get your fork and knife, and appreciate eating delicious healthy food while seeing the wellbeing and weight reduction benefits.

The Origin of Sirtfood Diet

A couple of health experts called Glen Matten and Aidan Goggins, whose spotlight has consistently been on smart dieting as opposed to weight reduction. In their new book The Sirtfood Diet, the pair spread out a feast plan which includes drinking three sirtfood green squeezes a day joined by adjusted sirtfood-rich meals, for example, a buckwheat and prawn stir-fry or smoked salmon sirt supersalad.

How It Is Better Than Other Diet

Sirtfoods are a recently found group of regular plant foods, known as sirtuin activators, which switch on our 'skinny' qualities – similar qualities enacted by fasting and exercise.

Unlike other diet plans, which are explicitly outfitted towards unhealthy and dramatic weight loss, the Sirtfood Diet is great if you essentially need to boost your resistant system, pack in certain nutrients and feel somewhat healthier.

Alongside this fat-burning impact, sirtfoods additionally have the unique capacity to - naturally control hunger and increase muscle function – making them the ideal answer for accomplishing a healthy weight.

Undoubtedly, their health-boosting impacts are incredible to such an extent that a few studies have shown them to be more powerful than professionally prescribed medications in forestalling constant infection, with apparent - benefits in diabetes, coronary illness and - Alzheimer's disease.

No big surprise cultures eating the most sirtfoods – including Italy and Japan – are the least fatty and most healthy on the planet. What's more, that is the reason we've formulated a diet based around them.

How the Sirt Food Diet Will Work For You

The sheer broadness of advantages that individuals have encountered has been a revelation, all accomplished by essentially putting together their diet concerning available and reasonable foods that a great many people as of now appreciate eating. What's more, that is all the Sirtfood Diet requires. It's tied in with receiving the rewards of regular foods that we were constantly intended to eat, but in the correct amounts and the right mixes to give us the body organization and prosperity we as a whole so profoundly need, and that can at last completely change us.

It doesn't expect you to perform extreme calorie limitation, nor does it demand grueling regimens (although remaining commonly dynamic is something worth being thankful for). What's more, the main bit of gear you'll require is a juicer. Also, not at all like each other diet out there that centers around what you ought to prohibit, the Sirtfood Diet centers around what you ought to incorporate.

To summarize everything, the Sirtfood Diet will support you:

• lose weight by burning fat, not muscle;

• burn fat, particularly from the stomach area, to fuel better health;

• prime your body for long term weight loss achievement;

• look and feel much improved and have more vitality;

• avoid suffering from severe calorie limitation or extraordinary craving;

• be liberated from grueling activity regimens;

• live a more extended, more advantageous, disease-free life.

STAGE 1 of the Sirt Food Diet

During the initial 3 days, calorie intake is confined to 1,000 calories (along these lines, still more than on a 5:2 fasting day). Sirt diet comprises of 3 Sirtfood-rich green juices and 1 Sirtfood-rich feast and two squares of dark chocolate.

During the remaining four days, calorie intake is expanded to 1, 500 calories, and every day the diet involves 2 Sirtfood-rich green juices and 2 Sirtfood-rich suppers.

During stage 1, you are not permitted to drink any liquor, yet you can freely drink water, tea, coffee, and green tea.

STAGE 2 of the Sirt Food Diet

Stage 2 doesn't concentrate on calorie limitation. Every day includes 3 Sirtfood-rich meals and one green juice, in addition to the alternative of 1 or 2 Sirtfood nibble snacks, whenever required.

In stage 2, you are permitted to drink red wine, however with some restraint (the suggestion is 2-3 glasses of red wine every week), just as water, tea, espresso, and green tea.

How It Is Better Than Other Diet

Sirtfoods are a recently found group of regular plant foods, known as sirtuin activators, which switch on our 'skinny' qualities – similar qualities enacted by fasting and exercise.

Unlike other diet plans, which are explicitly outfitted towards unhealthy and dramatic weight loss, the Sirtfood Diet is great if you essentially need to boost your resistant system, pack in certain nutrients and feel somewhat healthier.

Besides this fat-burning impact, sirtfoods have the unique capacity to -naturally control hunger and increase muscle function – making them the ideal answer for a healthy weight.

Undoubtedly, their health-boosting impacts are incredible to such an extent that a few studies have shown them to be more potent than professionally prescribed medications in forestalling constant infection, with apparent - benefits in diabetes, coronary illness, and - Alzheimer's disease.

No big surprise cultures eating the most sirtfoods – including Italy and Japan – are the least fatty and most healthy on the planet. What's more, that is the reason we've formulated a diet based around them.

Chapter 1

THE SCIENCE BEHIND IT SIRT FOOD DIET

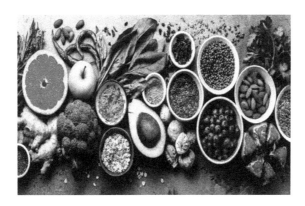

The Sirt food diet can't be named low-carb or low-fat. This diet is very not the same as its many forerunners while advocating numbers of very similar things: the ingestion of new, plant-based foods. As the name implies, this is a sirtuin based diet, yet what are sirtuins, and why have you never heard about them before?

There are seven sirtuin proteins – SIRT-1 to SIRT-71. They can be found all through your cells and the cells of each creature on the planet. Sirtuins are found in pretty much every living being and in pretty much all aspects of the cell, controlling what goes on. Supplement organization Elysium Health compares the body's cells to an office with sirtuins going about as the CEO, helping the cells respond to internal and external changes. They oversee what is done when it's set, and who does it.

Of the seven sirtuins, one work in your cell's cytoplasm, three in the cell's mitochondria, and another three in the cell's core. They have a wide number of jobs to perform, yet generally, they remove acetyl bunches from different proteins. These acetyl groups signal that the protein they are connected to is accessible to play out its capacity. Sirtuins evacuate the accessible flag and get the protein to utilize.

Sirtuins sound truly significant to your body's ordinary capacity, so for what reason is that you've never known about them?

The first sirtuin to be found was SIR2, a quality found during the 1970s which controlled the capacity of fruit flies to mate. It was until the 1990s that researchers discovered other, comparable proteins, in pretty much every type of life. Each living being had an alternate number of sirtuins –bacteria has one and yeast has five. Studies on mice show they have a similar number as humans, seven.

Sirtuins have been appeared to draw out life in yeast and mice. There is no proof of a similar impact in individuals, however, these sirtuins are available in pretty much every type of life, and many researchers are hopeful that if creatures as far separated as yeast and mice can see a similar impact from sirtuin activation; this may likewise extend to people.

For cells to work properly, our bodies need another substance called nicotinamide adenine dinucleotide. Elysium compares this substance to the cash an organization needs to continue working. Like any CEO, a sirtuin can stay with working appropriately if the cash flow is adequate. NAD+ was first found in 1906. You get you gracefully of NAD+ from your diet by eating foods made up of the building blocks of NAD+.

Fun Facts about Sirtuins:

1. Mice that have been designed to have elevated levels of SIRT-1 are both more dynamic and leaner than typical, while mice that need SIRT-1 inside and out are fatter and progressively inclined to different metabolic conditions.

2. Add the way that degrees of SIRT-1 is a lot of lower in obese individuals than in those of a "healthy" weight, and the case for the significance of sirtuins in weight loss gets convincing.

3. By creating a lasting change to your diet and adding the best Sirt foods to your eating plan, the creators of the Sirt food diet accept everybody can accomplish better health, all without losing muscle.

To Sum Up

Exercise and calorie limitation are the two sources of stress which urge our bodies to adjust to evolving conditions. If the pressure becomes too much, the outcome can be an injury. The body can even pass on, however at lower levels, we adjust, and this brief, low-level pressure is vital to many physiological changes.

For instance, weight on muscles, enough yet not all that much, is the thing that makes the body increase muscles.

So also, the creators of the Sirt food diet found that it is the point at which the body is worried, by exercise or low-calorie intake, that the impact of sirtuins kicks in, and it is this impact can be replicated by a diet rich in SIRT food.

Is this the diet for you?

Any diet plan you embrace includes some degree of cost and bother. It might likewise include risk. Anybody can write a diet book, as there is no compelling reason to have the diet restoratively affirmed. That is one motivation behind why all diet starts by recommending you consult a doctor. One thing you can do is take a look at the capabilities of the diet's creator.

The creators of the Sirt food diet are not TV characters or reality stars. They have certifiable logical information regarding the matter and both have Master's degrees to demonstrate it.

Aidan Goggins is a pharmacist, with a degree in a drug store and a Master's qualification in Nutritional Medicine. Glen Matten prepared at the Institute for Optimum Nutrition before finishing his Master's certificate in nourishing medication.

The Sirt food diet isn't their first joint effort. In 2012, they expressed "The Health Delusion," a book that assaulted a large number of the "long-held truths" of the diet and health industry. Therefore, they got the customer health book of the year grant by the Medical Journalists Association.

Having looked into the literature and posed the big question: "What might occur if we ate Sirtfoods? Would there be weight loss?" they went to ask: "What might happen to muscle, which is typically lost during practically any diet?"

To discover the appropriate responses, the creators directed a trail in an exclusive health spa close to London in the UK. There were 40 members. 39 finished the trial. Since the trial was done at a health spa, the creators had unlimited control over the food eaten by the members. Note this isn't generally the situation in "medical" trials where the members report what they ate.

The revelation and history of sirtuins

There were various amounts of sirtuins in each animal. For example, yeast has five sirtuins, microscopic life forms have one, mice have seven, and individuals have seven.

The way that sirtuins were found across species infers they were "saved" with advancement. Characteristics that are "proportioned" have comprehensive limits in various or all species. What was now to be known, however, was the methods by which noteworthy sirtuins would wind up being.

In 1991, Elysium individual advocate and MIT researcher Leonard Guarente, close by graduated class understudies Nick Austriaco and Brian Kennedy, drove trials to all the almost certain to perceive how yeast developed. By some incident, Austriaco endeavored to create social orders of various yeast strains from tests he had taken care of in his ice chest for a seriously long time, which made an upsetting space for the strains. Only a segment of these strains could create from here, yet Guarente and his group recognized a model: The strains of yeast that persevere through the best in the cooler were in like manner the longest-lived. This provided guidance to Guarente so he could focus solely on these long-living strains of yeast.

This provoked the distinguishing proof of SIR2 as a quality that advanced life span in yeast. It's basic to note more research is required on SIR2's possessions in individuals. The Guarantee lab thus found that ousting SIR2 contracted yeast life go fundamentally, while specifically, extending the amount of copies of the SIR2 quality from one to two extended the existence length in yeast. Regardless, what started SIR2 ordinarily by and by couldn't appear to be found.

This is the place acetyl bundles become conceivably the most significant factor. It was from the first thought that SIR2 might be a deacetylating protein — which implies it removed those acetyl groups— from various atoms, yet no one knew whether this was substantial since all endeavors to show this development in a test tube exhibited negative. Guarantee and his group had the alternative to find that SIR2 in yeast could just deacetylate various proteins inside seeing the coenzyme NAD+, nicotinamide adenine dinucleotide.

In Guarente's own words: "Without NAD+, SIR2 sits inactive. That was the fundamental finding on the round portion of sirtuin science."

Power of Sirtfood

The Sirtfood Diet's authors make bold claims, including that the diet will induce super-charge weight loss, turn the "skinny gene" on, and prevent disease.

The thing is they don't have any evidence to back them up.

Up to date, there is no evidence that the Sirtfood Diet has a more beneficial effect on weight loss than any other diet limited by calories.

Also, albeit huge numbers of those nourishments have healthy properties, no drawn-out human examinations have been conducted to decide if eating a diet rich in sirt nourishments has any substantial health advantages. However, a pilot study completed by the writers and involving 39 members from their fitness center is accounted for in the Sirtfood Diet book. Be that as it may, the aftereffects of this study doesn't appear to have been published elsewhere.

Participants followed the diet for a week and were walking every day. At the weekend, participants lost a total of 7 pounds (3.2 kg) and retained or even added muscle mass.

Those findings, however, are hardly shocking. Limiting your calorie intake to 1,000 calories, and actively exercising, would almost always induce weight loss.

Regardless, this form of rapid weight loss is neither permanent nor long-lasting, and this research did not monitor participants beyond the first week to see whether they gained any of the weight back, as is normally the case.

As well as consuming fat and muscle, when the body is drained of energy, it uses its emergency energy reserves or glycogen.

Every glycogen molecule requires 3–4 water molecules for storage. If your body uses glycogen, the water always gets rid of it. It is known as "weight in water."

Only about one-third of the weight-loss comes from fat during the first week of extreme calorie restriction, while the other two-thirds come from water, muscle, and glycogen.

As soon as your calorie consumption increases, your body refills its glycogen stores, and the weight comes right back.

Unfortunately, this kind of calorie restriction can likewise cause your body to lower its metabolic rate, causing you to need even fewer calories daily for energy than before.

The sirt diet may help you lose a few pounds; however, it might come back as soon as you stop it.

As well as consuming fat and muscle, when the body is drained of energy, it uses its emergency energy reserves or glycogen.

Each glycogen molecule requires 3–4 water molecules for storage. If your body uses glycogen, the water always gets rid of it. It is known as "weight in water."

Pretty much 33% of the weight reduction originates from fat during the first week of extreme calorie limitation, while 66% originate from skin, glycogen, and muscle.

Your body will replenish its glycogen stores as soon as your calorie intake increases, and the weight returns right back.

Unfortunately, this sort of calorie limitation can likewise make your body decrease its metabolic rate, causing energy requirements to be even lower in calories per day.

This diet is likely to help you lose a few pounds in the beginning, but it'll probably return as soon as the diet is done.

As far as disease prevention is concerned, it is likely three weeks not long enough to have any meaningful long-term effects.

On the other hand, it might very well be smart to add sirtfood to your daily diet over the long term. But you might as well miss the diet in that scenario, and start doing it now.

This eating regimen can help you get thinner since it is low in calories. However, when the diet finishes, the weight is probably going to return. The diet is too short even to consider impacting on your health over the long haul.

The Remarkable Results

The Sirtfood Diet was tested by forty and finished by thirty-nine individuals at XK. Of these thirty-nine, two in the trial were stout, fifteen were overweight, and twenty-two had an ordinary/healthy body index (BMI). The study had a genuinely even gender split, with twenty-one ladies and eighteen men. Being individuals from a health club, before they began, they were bound to practice and know about proper dieting than everybody.

A trick of many diets is to utilize a heavily overweight and undesirable example of individuals to show the advantages, as from the outset, they shed pounds the fastest and most drastically, basically lightening up the diet outcomes. Our rationale was the inverse: if we got great results with this moderately healthy group, it would set the least benchmark of what was attainable.

The outcomes far surpassed our effectively exclusive requirements. Results were predictable and astounding: a normal 7 pounds of weight loss in seven days in the wake of representing muscle gain.

As though that weren't sufficient, we saw something different much progressively great, which was the sort of weight loss. Regularly, when individuals get fit, they will lose some fat yet they will likewise lose some muscle—this is not all bad about eating fewer carbs. We were shocked to locate the inverse. Our members either kept up their muscles or picked up muscle. As we will discover later in the book, this is a vastly increasingly great sort of weight loss, and an extraordinary element of the Sirtfood Diet.

No member neglected to see improvements in body structure. What's more, recollect, the entirety of this was accomplished without dietary hardship or overwhelming activity regimens.

This is what we found:

• Participants accomplished surprising and quick outcomes, losing a normal of 7 pounds in seven days.

• Weight loss was generally perceptible around the stomach area.

• Rather than being lost, the muscle was either kept up or increased.

• Participants once in a while, felt hungry.

• Participants felt an expanded feeling of imperativeness and well-being.

• Participants announced looking better and more advantageous.

Not All Vegetables and Fruits Are Made Equal

Since 1986 two of the biggest nourishing studies in US history have been attempted simultaneously by scientists at Harvard University: the Health Professionals Follow-Up Study, inspecting men's dietary habits and health, and the Nurses' Health Study, exploring the equivalent for females. Drawing on this vast wealth of data, specialists investigated the connection between the dietary habits for more than 124,000 individuals and changes in body weight over a twenty-four-year period finishing off with 2011.

They discovered something exceptional. As a feature of a standard American diet, expending certain plant foods fought off weight gain, yet devouring others had no impact by any means. What was the distinction between them? Everything came down to whether the foods were wealthy in particular kinds of regular plant chemicals known as polyphenols. We about all will in general put on weight as we age, yet devouring higher measures of polyphenols had eminent effect in forestalling this. When analyzed in more prominent detail, just specific kinds of polyphenols stood apart as being successful for keeping people slim, the analysts found. Among those successful were similar groups of normal plant chemicals concoctions that the pharmaceutical business was angrily attempting to transform into a marvel pill for their capacity to turn on our sirtuin qualities.

The end was significant: not all plant foods (counting leafy foods vegetables) are equivalent with regards to controlling our weight. Rather, we have to begin researching plant foods for their polyphenol content, and afterward thusly examine the capacity of those polyphenols to turn on our "skinny" sirtuin qualities. This is an extreme thought that contradicts the predominant creed of our occasions. The time has come to relinquish the nonexclusive, blanket that advises us to eat two cups of foods grown from the ground and a half cups of vegetables daily as a major aspect of a balanced diet. We need just check out us to perceive how little effect that has had.

With this move in judging how plant foods are beneficial for us, some skinny differences got evident. The many foods that alleged health specialists cautioned us away from, for example, chocolate, coffee, and tea, are in reality so rich in sirtuin-activating polyphenols that they trump most fruits and vegetables out there. How often do we scowl as we swallow our vegetables since we're informed that is the proper activity, possibly to feel regretful if we even look at that after-supper chocolate treat? A definitive incongruity is that cocoa is perhaps the best food we might be eating. Its utilization has now been shown to enact sirtuin qualities, with different benefits for controlling body weight by consuming fat, decreasing appetite, and improving muscle function. And that is before we assess its large number of other medical advantages, a greater amount of which to come later.

In complete we have distinguished twenty foods rich in polyphenols that have been appeared to enact our sirtuin qualities, and together this structure the premise of the Sirtfood Diet. While the story began with red wine as the first Sirtfood, we currently realize these other nineteen foods either match or trump it for their sirtuin-enacting polyphenol content. Just as cocoa, these incorporate other notable and much-delighted in foods, for example, additional virgin olive oil, red onions, garlic, parsley, chilies, kale, strawberries, walnuts, escapades, tofu, green tea, and even coffee. While every food has amazing health accreditations of its own, as we are going to see, the genuine magic happens when we join these foods to make an entire diet.

A Common Link Among the World's Healthiest Diets

As we study further, we found that the best sources of Sirtfoods were found in the diet of those experiencing the lowest rates of sickness and obesity in the world. From the Kuna American Indians, who seem immune to hypertension and show low rates of obesity, diabetes, cancer, and early death. Because of an incredibly rich intake of the Sirtfood cocoa; to Okinawa, Japan, where a smorgasbord of Sirtfoods, smooth figures, and long life all go hand in hand. To India, where the ravenous craving for all things spicy, particularly the Sirtfood turmeric, has left cancer in its wake.

However, the diet is the jealousy of the remainder of the Western world, a conventional Mediterranean diet, where the advantages of Sirtfoods genuinely stick out. Here corpulence just doesn't win and interminable sickness is the special case, not the standard. Additional virgin olive oil, wild leafy greens, nuts, berries, red wine, dates, and herbs are generally powerful Sirtfoods, and all feature prominently in the local Mediterranean diet. The logical world has been left in awe considering the latest agreement that following a Mediterranean diet is more viable than checking calories for weight loss, and more powerful than pharmaceutical medications for halting the disease.

This carries us to PREDARKED, a game-changing study of the Mediterranean diet, distributed in 2013. It was directed on right around 7,400 people at high risk of cardiovascular sickness, and the outcomes were acceptable to such an extent that the trial was halted ahead of schedule—after only five years. The reason for PREDARKED was flawlessly basic. It asked what the distinction would be between a Mediterranean-style diet enhanced with either additional virgin olive oil or nuts (particularly walnuts) and a progressively traditional cutting edge diet. Furthermore, what a distinction it was. The adjustment in diet reduced the rate of cardiovascular infection by around 30 percent, an outcome medicate organizations can just dream of. Upon further development, it was discovered that there was additionally a 30 percent fall in diabetes, alongside noteworthy drops in aggravation, enhancements in memory and brain health, and an enormous 40 percent reduction in corpulence, with eminent fat loss, particularly around the stomach area.

However, at first scientists couldn't clarify what created these emotional advantages. Neither the measures of calories, fats, and sugars are eaten—the run of the mill estimates used to survey the food we eat—nor physical movement levels contrasted between the groups to clarify the discoveries. There must be something different going on.

Then the eureka moment struck. Both additional virgin olive oil and walnuts stand apart for their excellent substance of sirtuin-enacting polyphenols. Basically, by adding these in critically adding up to an ordinary Mediterranean diet, what the analysts had accidentally made was a superrich Sirtfood diet. They found that it conveyed amazing outcomes.

So analysts breaking down PREDARKED thought of a cunning theory. If it is the polyphenols that at last issue, they considered, at that point the individuals who ate the greater part of them would encounter their total advantages by living the longest. So they ran the details, and the results were staggering. Over only five years, the individuals who expended the most elevated levels of polyphenols had 37 percent fewer deaths compared with the individuals who ate the least.[10] Intriguingly, this is twofold the reduction in mortality that treatment with the most generally recommended blockbuster statin drugs is found to bring. At long last we had the clarification for the awe-inspiring advantages this study observed, and it was more remarkable than any drug in presence.

The analysts likewise noted something different of significance. While many studies have recently discovered that individual Sirtfoods give great medical advantages, they were never significant enough to broaden life. PREDARKED was the first of its sort. The thing that matters was that it took a look at an example of foods as opposed to a single food. Various foods give diverse sirtuin-initiating polyphenols, which work in agreement to create a considerably more remarkable result than any single food can. This left us with an unstoppable end. Genuine health isn't harvested through one single supplement or even one "wonder food." What you need is an entire diet loaded up with a blend of Sirtfoods all working in cooperative energy. Also, this is the thing that prompted the formation of the Sirtfood Diet.

Chapter 2

THE "SKINNY GENE"

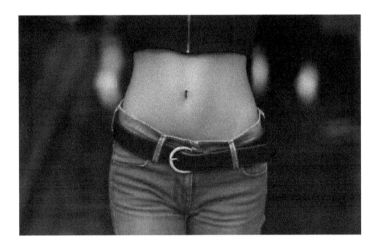

The ALK (anaplastic lymphoma kinase) quality is the variation that encourages protection from weight gain, regardless of what diet an individual has. It diminishes individuals stay thin, possibly opening another frontier in medicines for weight.

The gene assumes a role in resisting weight gain in the metabolically healthy, slight individuals. It is found in the nerve center, the area in the brain answerable for controlling hunger and how an individual controls fat.

The ALK quality makes a protein called anaplastic lymphoma kinase, which is associated with cell growth. The quality is likewise connected to specific diseases and distinguished as a driver of tumor growth.

ALK Variations

The group broke down the DNA of more than 47,000 individuals between the ages of 20 and 44 years of age. They took a look at the data from Estonia's biobank, an organic database gathered from a huge level of the Estonian population.

The analysts recognized thin, healthy people in the most minimal sixth percentile of weight. The benchmark group, then again, were those in the 30th and 50th percentile. Individuals from the 95th percentile were labeled as the obese group. The group distinguished the variations of qualities that seemed to happen all the more frequently in the thin group.

In the wake of examining the database, the group found that a few variations in the ALK quality were attached to low defenselessness to weight gain in normally dainty individuals. The group likewise found that erasing the quality had prompted more slender flies. Further, mice hereditarily changed to do not have the ALK quality additionally demonstrated stamped protection from weight.

Therapeutics Targeting the Gene

The group says that therapeutics focusing on the gene may assist researchers with handling and battle stoutness later on. If there could be an approach to close down the ALK quality or lessen its capacity, at any rate, individuals can remain thin. At present, ALK medicines, for example, inhibitors are being utilized in cancer.

Further research is expected to check whether tranquilize inhibitors are successful for this reason before they are trialed in people. The group anticipates the second phase of the study, which means to compare the discoveries and biobank records on the health, DNA, and movement levels of different populaces over the globe.

The group additionally plans to concentrate on how neurons that express the ALK direct the mind at an atomic level to adjust metabolism and advance thinness.

The advancement came when we found that the advantages of fasting were interceded by activating our ancient sirtuin qualities, otherwise called the "skinny gene". At the point when energy is hard to find, precisely as found in calorie limitation, an expanded measure of pressure is put on our cells. This is detected by the sirtuins, which at that point get turned on and communicate amazing signs that fundamentally adjust how our cells act.

Sirtuins ramp up metabolism, increment the effectiveness of muscles, switch on fat consumption, lessen inflammation and fix any harm in cells. As a result, sirtuins make us fitter, less fatty and more beneficial.

Are The Skinny Gene A Thing

Throughout the years, different research trials have been directed to help decide whether there are extremely 'skinny genes. For what reason do a few people truly battle with their weight though others appear to eat what they need without gaining any additional weight? While diet and way of life are the undeniable contributing components, weight differences in animals have given us the motivation to accept there might be more to it than that; and maybe there's likewise a greater amount of an inward driving variable - genes.

Throughout the years, up to 50 different genes have been discovered which are without a doubt thought to have an impact on our weight and body piece. Huge numbers of these are expected to impact how we ingest and use fats, and even have an impact on our appetite.

One of the latest revelations was the 'skinny gene' which has been alleged 'adipose'[1]. This was initially found in natural fruit flies, yet has additionally been found in rodents and people. If the quality is turned on, the individual is bound to be 'skinny', while if it's turned off, we're bound to store progressively fat, or fat tissue. In any case, strangely the 'skinny gene' isn't believed to be just turned on or off, however it might be turned on to fluctuating degrees in various people.

The Role of Gut Bacteria

Just as inalienable genes having an impact on our body weight, there are possibly other inside impacts as well, for example, the balance of bacteria in our gut.

Gut bacteria preliminaries have demonstrated that the pervasiveness of particular kinds of microbes is connected to various body loads among people[2], and although it's not surely known how precisely these functions, we realize that these microorganisms can discharge synthetic chemicals which can conceivably adjust our genes too.

Although gut microorganisms can be affected from birth (with cesarean conceived babies found to have an alternate equalization from those conceived normally), there are a lot of steps you can take as far as your diet and way of life to help advance a healthier balance of gut bacteria and, accordingly, possibly impact your weight thusly as well – another significant thought!

The Influence of Diet

Although individuals are getting increasingly intrigued by genetics and what genes we may or not have –you're left with your genetic makeup. In any case, what I truly need to pressure is that you can impact these genes in various manners:

1 - The Power of Nourishment Could Turn Genes On Or Off

We realize that diet and our condition can impact our genes straightforwardly. Strikingly the 'skinny gene' is believed to be turned on to various degrees in various individuals – so everybody has it, we simply need to impact it.

2 - Genetic Components Aren't the Most Important Thing in The World

Although certain individuals might be pre-arranged to specific things because of their genes, with regards to bodyweight (and loads of different factors, for example, disease states), there are heaps of motivation to accept that we can defeat even genes, because of outside impacts, for example, diet and way of life, at any rate to a limited degree! For by far most individuals, dealing with their diet or taking a shot at more exercise will have the desired impact when done perfectly.

3 - Genes Alone Aren't to Be Faulted For The Ongoing Increment In Weight

Just accusing our genes risks being somewhat of a cop-out with regards to body weight. As both corpulence and the related illnesses, for example, diabetes has expanded exponentially in all pieces of the world over a similar time frame in recent years, we realize that genes aren't the entire story. This pattern proposes diet, dietary patterns and social impacts are substantially more liable to assume the primary job.

Are There Explicit Diets That Can Impact Our 'Skinny Genes'?

There is by all accounts a consistent flow of new craze diets accessible these days and it very well may be hard to tell which, if any of them, are probably going to be appropriate for supporting your health or explicit weight reduction goals.

Regarding conceivably impacting that ' skinny gene' the Sirtfood Diet has been given some uncommon consideration as of late. The Sirtfood Diet is alleged because it is wealthy in nourishments high in exceptional chemical compound called sirtuin activators. Sirtuins are a particular class of compounds which are thought to have useful impacts in the body and the nourishments they can be found in incorporate bunches of healthy things, for example, green tea, dull chocolate, citrus natural products, apples, turmeric, blueberries, kale, and red wine.

Presently, although I'm supportive of remembering these nourishments for your diet, it must be stated, the exploration is somewhat crude regarding the particular impacts that these food sources can have, because of their sirtuin activator content. The Sirtfood Diet rules are commonly truly controlled, genuinely severe with no place for breathing space, they include cutting calories drastically and substituting appropriate dinners for juices. Although these sorts of plans can now and again be useful in the present moment for instance, as a feature of a delicate detox, longer-term it's probably not going to be so maintainable. It's significantly more reasonable to embrace a way of life which underpins your health and body weight in the long term.

Summarizing and Making A Move

In this way, in case you're frantic to make a move and bolster a more beneficial you, skinny genes or not, here's my recommendation:

1 – Incorporate the Sirtfood Diet Parts Into Your Diet At Any Rate

Instead of following an overly severe system and prescriptive recipes, why not simply put forth an attempt to incorporate a greater amount of the components of the Sirtfood diet in your system at any rate? Regardless of whether the sirtuins are having explicit activities in the body, these nourishments are stuffed brimming with nutrients, minerals, and antioxidants which are significant for supporting healthy substantial procedures and a buzzing metabolism.

I truly accept that cooking from new is the way into a healthy body weight. It's all the prepared nourishments with concealed sugars, salts, fat (and the rest!) that are considerably more liable to add to us heaping on the pounds. Eat new, start arranging and preparing your dinners and you'll before long feel and notice the distinction.

2 – Don't Disregard the Solid Fats

Something that the Sirtfood diet is ostensibly missing is a decent portion of healthy fats. Individuals are frequently prone to avoid fats, particularly when attempting to shed pounds, yet in all honesty, we need healthy fats to help our digestion and remain lean!

An ongoing report likewise featured this idea and found that older individuals who effectively presented an extra 300 calories for each day from walnuts had no negative impacts on body weight or body piece which incorporates fat dispersion. This is truly encouraging, and simply think about the potential outcomes if you incorporated these and cut out something less accommodating! So no reason, get consolidating those fats!

3 – Regardless of Your Qualities, Assume   Responsibility For Your Way Of Life

Indeed, even the specialists have concurred that there's nothing you can't do to impact your genes. So regardless of whether we are inclined to certain body types or disease states, it just methods we are at more danger of these various states, it isn't unavoidable that we'll get influenced. Subsequently, our diet, every day propensities, and way of life variables would all be able to have an impact and even little changes might have the universe of effect.

One top tip to consider is how much water you drink. We realize that water impacts each arrangement of our body, and research has recommended that this basic constituent of our diet could be urgent for supporting our qualities and by and large health.

Not exclusively are the advantages of water there, however, if you drink more water you're more averse to drink different things – other conceivably progressively harmful things. There's been a consistent increment in the utilization of calorific beverages as of late, and with calories come all the sugar, fake sugars, caffeine, and liquor which are normal segments of beverages that aren't water – all of which aren't probably going to help your digestion! In this way, drink up, and include a cut of lemon or some other organic product in case you're battling at first.

4 – Herbal Partners

In case you're attempting to get in shape, although there's not prone to be any handy solution as far as products (yes individuals, diet and way of life truly is critical!) there are a couple of zones you could focus on to help your advancement:

Support your metabolism with Kelp;

Supporting your thyroid organ and digestion is consistently a significant thought in case you're chipping away at your weight. Particularly in the way to deal with menopause, or if your hormones have been playing up as of late, your thyroid may require some delicate help and our Kelp tablets with a reasonable portion of iodine can be an invite expansion!

Bolster Your Stomach With Unpleasant Herbs

Supporting your stomach with some severe herbs, for example, Yarrow guarantees that you are retaining all the basic supplements from your food and benefiting as much as possible from them. Magnesium helps bolster insulin affectability and B nutrients help us to change over our food into energy– these are only two supplements worth referencing which are excessively significant for supporting a healthy body weight.

Bolster Your Gut with Prebiotics

All together for the bacteria in your gut to endure and carry out their responsibility adequately (metabolism is a major piece of this), they should be in an appropriate domain. Including a decent portion of L+ lactic corrosive to you day by day system by utilizing Molkosan can help make only that, and you'll unquestionably need to do this first before considering presenting any probiotics supplements.

The Change to Sirtfoods

"Sirtfoods" are the notable methods for enacting our sirtuin genes in the most ideal manner. These are the marvel nourishments especially rich in explicit regular plant chemicals, called polyphenols, which can address our sirtuin genes, turning them on. They emulate the impacts of fasting and practice and in doing so bring amazing advantages by helping the body to all the more likely control glucose levels, consume fat, form muscle, and lift health and memory.

Since they're fixed, plants have built up an exceptionally advanced stress-reaction system and produce polyphenols to assist them with adjusting to the difficulties of their condition. At the point when we devour these plants, we likewise expend these polyphenol supplements. Their impact is significant: they enact our natural pressure reaction pathways.

While all plants have pressure reaction frameworks, just certain ones have created to deliver essential measures of sirtuin-actuating polyphenols. These plants are Sirt foods. Their revelation implies that rather than severe diets or burdensome exercise programs, there's currently a progressive better approach to actuate your sirtuin qualities: eating a diet inexhaustible in Sirt foods. The best part is that this one includes putting (Sirt)foods onto your plate, not taking them off.

Chapter 3

FAT LOSS VS MUSCLE LOSS

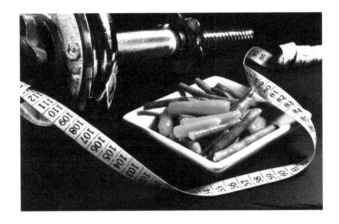

Fat Loss vs Weight Loss: It's Not The Same.

People say they want to shed some pounds. The thing is, "weight" can be a few different things. For instance:

People frequently say they want to get in shape. This thing is, "weight" can be a couple of various things. For instance:

- Muscle.

- Fat.

- Glycogen.

- Poop.

- Water.

If all you care about is losing weight, you might get food poisoning and poop your brains out, or sit in a sauna and sweat a great deal. You could remove a leg and you'll lose "weight" fine and dandy. (Disclaimer: please do not do that).

However, If you are reading this, I will accept that you would prefer not to lose any of this other stuff. Or maybe, what you need to do here is lose fat, NOT muscle.

How Fat Loss Happens

Loss of fat has only one significant necessity: a caloric shortage.

A caloric deficit or shortage is the state when you expend fewer calories than your body consumes for vitality.

When this occurs, it powers your body to locate an elective wellspring of vitality to consume for fuel rather, and that will principally wind up being your stored body fat.

How Muscle Loss Occurs

Ideally, the ONLY thing your body would burn while in a caloric shortage is your stored body fat.

In any case, it turns out there's a subsequent vitality source available: your muscle tissue.

And keeping in mind that you may need your body to just burn fat and not burn any muscle at all, actually, your body doesn't generally give a crap about what you desire.

All it thinks about is keeping you alive (fun actuality: your body can not tell if you're in a caloric shortage because you are trying to lose some fat, or because you are at risk of starving to death), and to get that going, it will need to take some stored energy/vitality from somewhere.

That can mean muscle, fat, or a mix of both.

How to Prevent It.

What you have to do here is change your diet and exercise in ways that will cause your body more likely to burn body fat, and less likely to burn muscle fat.

How do you do this, you ask?

Here are the eight best ways to lose fat without losing muscle:

1. Eat A Sufficient Amount of Protein

Your total daily protein consumption is the most significant dietary factor when it comes to maintaining muscle.

It's not specific food decisions, or when you eat, or how regularly you eat, or supplements, or carbs, or even the specific size of your caloric deficiency.

Healthfully, the greatest key to losing fat without losing muscle is eating an adequate amount of protein every day.

Even without a legitimate weight training routine, a greater amount of the weight you lose will be muscle mass because of a higher protein consumption.

Along these lines, the initial step to any muscle-preserving diet will eat a perfect measure of protein constantly.   How much is that precisely? Indeed, given the available research...

For most individuals, between the range of 0.8 – 1.3g of protein per pound of your present body weight is the sweet spot for preserving muscle during fat loss.

2. Increase or Maintain Strength Levels

Would you be amazed if I disclosed to you that utilizing a very much structured weight training program is essential for losing fat while maintaining muscle?

No? I didn't think so.

What may amaze you, however, is that it's more than simply "utilizing an exercise program" or "doing strength training" that gives the muscle-holding benefits we desire.

The primary training boost for building muscle is dynamic strain overload, which implies bit by bit getting more grounded over time.

For instance, if you lift some weights for the same number of reps for the following 20 years, your body will still have no reason to build extra muscle. However, if you gradually lift the same weight for more reps, or lift more weight, your body would then have more reason to build more muscle.

What's more, this same idea applies to keeping up muscle also. You will probably give your body a reason to maintain the muscle mass it already has.

How do you do that?

At least, aim to maintain your present strength levels all through the length of the weight loss program, or, if conceivable, increment them. Doing so gives a "muscle support" signal that tells your body it needs to maintain the muscle it has or build more.

Consider it like this. When your body is searching for an alternative fuel source to consume for vitality, and it can pick muscle mass or body fat for that reason, it will be more averse to pick muscle (and bound to pick fat) if it sees there is a reason behind keeping the muscle around.

3. Try not to Reduce Calories By Too Much

As I clarified before, a caloric shortage should be available with the goal for you to lose body fat, and that implies you're going to need to diminish your calorie consumption to some degree.

The thing is, that level of shortage can be a wide range of various sizes going from pointlessly little to too much.

And keeping in mind that diverse deficit sizes can suit certain individuals in specific circumstances more so than others, research and certifiable experience fit toward a moderate deficiency being perfect for some, reasons, including preserving muscle.

Specifically...

The perfect caloric deficiency for the vast majority is between 15-25% beneath their maintenance level, with an even 20 percent regularly being a decent beginning stage.

In this way, for instance, if your upkeep level happened to be 2500 calories and you needed to make a 20 percent deficiency, you'd aim to eat around 2000 calories every day.

Why Not Use A Larger Deficit?

This is the moment that you might be asking why a bigger shortage isn't being utilized. All things considered, wouldn't diminish your calories by more than this make weight loss happen significantly quicker?

That is correct, it surely would.

However, remember this isn't just about "weight loss." Our objective is more explicit than that. We need to lose fat... and do it without losing muscle.

What's more, for that reason, enormous shortages, low-calorie diets, and "quick" weight loss will be bad ideas for many people.

Indeed, this kind of thing is an impractical notion for some reasons, as it can worsen:

- Hormonal adaptations.
- Hunger
- Mood
- Metabolic Slowdown
- Sleep Quality
- Water Retention
- Fatigue and Lethargy
- Recovery and Performance
- Reproductive Function and Libido
- Sustainability and Adherence
- Disordered Eating Habits.

4. Decrease Weight Training Frequency And/Or Frequency

A caloric shortage is a vitality shortage, and keeping in mind that this is awesome (and required) for losing any measure of body fat, it's not perfect for boosting weight training recuperation and performance.

This is something we just discussed a second prior as far as bigger deficits having a bigger negative effect in such manner.

However, even with only a moderate deficit set up, there is probably going to still be some drop-off in recuperation/performance contrasted with when you're at maintenance or in an overflow.

Why does this matter, you ask?

Since the exercise routine you were (or would be) utilizing with extraordinary accomplishment for an objective like building muscle under non-deficit conditions presently can be a lot for your body to deal with in the energy-deficient state it is in currently.

Also, that sort of situation? That is what makes strength to be lost. What's more, when strength is lost in a deficiency, muscle loss is what ordinarily follows.

If you're utilizing an exercise routine that includes more volume (reps, sets, and works out) or potentially recurrence (exercises every week) than you can handle, you may see things getting more difficult for you, or see that you're getting weaker, or that reps are diminishing, or that progress is relapsing, or that weight on the bar should be decreased, and in the end... that muscle is being lost.

How to Prevent It

How do you avoid all of this?

This could mean decreasing training volume (for example doing somewhat fewer sets), decreasing training volume (for example utilizing a 3-day exercise routine rather than a 5-day exercise routine), or a blend of both.

The specific changes you should make (or whether any modifications really should be made at this stage) relies upon the particular exercise routine you're utilizing and your recuperation capabilities.

5. Get Pre And Post Workout Nutrition Right

Your pre and post-workout/exercise meals, otherwise known as the meals you eat before and after your session, are not exactly as very significant as the vast majority portray them.

They are only one of numerous components of your diet that are auxiliary to your all-out calorie and macronutrient consumption (for example fat, protein, and carbs), which is consistently what makes a difference most with regards to losing fat or maintaining/building muscle.

Having said that, your pre and post-workout meals matter still.

No, they are not capable of breaking or making your success, but they are capable of giving advantages that can improve your exhibition during an exercise, and upgrade recuperation related training adjustments after an exercise.

What's more, since we know that 1) recovery and performance are diminished to a certain level while we're in a deficiency, and 2) this can expand the danger of muscle loss... it's quite safe to state that these are benefits we need to get.

Anyway, what do you have to do to get them?

Expend a decent amount of carbs and protein within one to two hours before and after your workout/exercises.

6. Incorporate Calorie or Refeeds Cycling

As I've clarified all through this chapter, the basic act of being in a drawn-out caloric shortage or deficit makes an assortment of changes happen that expand the danger of muscle loss.

From hormonal adjustments, to expanded fatigue and lethargy, to a decrease in recuperation and performance... it all makes losing muscle-bound to occur.

Luckily for us, there are strategies we can use to help limit these impacts or possibly even reverse them.

These strategies include:

• Calorie Cycling

• Refeeds

• Diet Breaks

Refeeds and calorie cycling permit us to briefly stop our shortage by deliberately eating more calories – particularly from carbs, as carbs have the greatest positive effect on a hormone called leptin – to get back up to our maintenance level or into an excess.

In addition to being valuable from the angle of making your diet progressively sustainable, these strategies will likewise serve to recharge muscle glycogen stores (which assists with performance and strength) and positively affect various psychological and physiological factors that are contrarily affected during a shortage or deficit.

• Refeeds

Refeeds can be done a couple of various ways, however, it's a 24 hour time of being out of your shortage and eating somewhere close level and 500 calories above it (with the expansion in calories coming principally through carbs). I have discovered one refeed day per each week as a decent frequency for those with a normal measure of fat to lose, and once every other week is useful for those with an above-average amount to lose.

• Calorie Cycling

Calorie cycling is numerous refeed days (for instance 2-3) over seven days, often arranged so that you are taking more calories on your exercise days, and less calories on your rest days, with the particular daily amount balanced varying to still have the proposed total weekly net shortage/deficit at long last.

Along these lines, with an average weight loss diet, you would be devouring about the same amount of macronutrients and calories constantly, and be in a steady caloric shortage day after day.

Refeeds and calorie cycling change this by embeddings non-deficit days to help diminish the negative impacts a prolonged deficit can have, and make us bound to retain muscle while losing fat.

7. Take Diet Breaks When Needed

Take what we just talked about refeeds and calorie cycling, however, envision their positive advantages being more significant.

Imagine that as opposed to diminishing the negative impacts of a prolonged deficit, we could reverse those impacts to some level.

That is the full diet break.

A diet break is commonly a one to two-week time-frame where you come out of the deficit and back up to your maintenance level with the end goal of quickly permitting many of the things that suck about fat loss. (for example metabolic and hormonal adaptations) to recoup a piece and return to normal (or possibly, closer to normal).

This is advantageous for some reasons, one of which is forestalling muscle loss.

How To Do It

To take a diet break, increment your calorie consumption (essentially through extra carbs) with the goal that you are at your maintenance level each day for a time of one to two weeks.

Diet break frequency ought to be reliant on personal preferences/needs, and how much fat you need to lose. Generally, once every six to sixteen weeks tend to be perfect for most (maybe every 6-12 weeks if you have less to lose, and each ten to sixteen weeks if you have more to lose).

Much the same as with refeeds and calorie cycling, diet breaks are likewise a major piece of my Superior Fat Loss program.

8. Avoid Excessive Amounts of Cardio

Cardio is extra exercise... and extra exercise requires extra recuperation.

While this can be dangerous at any time and under any circumstance, we realize the potential is higher when we're in the energy insufficient (and recuperation-impaired) state we should be in for fat loss to happen. Which we are.

This implies, the more workout we do, the more danger we posture to our capacity to adequately recoup, both regarding the body parts being utilized the most (regularly the legs with most types of cardio), just as the central nervous system (CNS)... which influences everything.

Furthermore, if recuperation starts to suffer, performance and strength will suffer. What's more, when performance and strength suffer, so will your capacity to assemble or maintain muscle while losing fat.

Precisely how much of an effect cardio has in such manner is difficult to state, as it relies upon the specific duration, intensity, and frequency of the activity being finished.

For instance...

• Three cardio sessions every week will have less of an effect than five to seven sessions.

• Thirty minutes of cardio will have less of an effect than one hour to two hours.

• A low-intensity activity – like strolling – would have next to zero effect contrasted with a more moderate-intensity activity, for example, jogging.

• And neither would have nearly as quite a bit of an effect as something with a high intensity – like HIIT (high-intensity interval training, for example, running) – which can nearly be like adding weight training exercise as far as the pressure and stress it puts on your body and how recovery-intensive it is.

Farewell Fat, Hello Muscle!

There you have it... the best things you can do to guarantee you lose fat without losing muscle simultaneously.

While the initial two things (adequate protein consumption and keeping up/expanding strength) are the most significant, most logically bolstered, and generally beneficial in this regard, I've discovered that actualizing the entirety of the recommendations in this book is what produces the best outcomes.

Chapter 4

SIRTFOOD DIET HEALTH BENEFITS

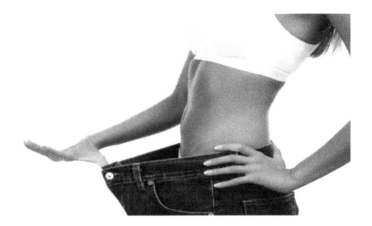

There is proof that sirtuin activators provide a wide variety of health benefits like muscle strengthening and appetite suppression. Or improved memory, better control of blood sugar level, and the clearance of damage caused by free radical molecules that build up in cells and result in cancer and other diseases. Let's have a look in detail at the main benefits the Sirtfood Diet will guarantee you for a lifetime.

Immediate Weight Loss

The most obvious of the health benefit is that you will lose weight on this diet. Whether you are exercising or not, there is no way that you would not lose weight when you follow the diet to a T. This diet will have you restrict your calories enough that anyone would lose weight. The average person uses around 2,000 calories per day; you will be providing yourself with 1,000 or 1,500 calories based on the phase that you are in.

Weight loss is caused by a calorie deficit — it is as simple as that. When you restrict your calories, but you keep your metabolism up, you will find that you will naturally lose weight.

Appetite under Control

Though your first few days on Sirtfood Diet you may find that you are ravenous as your body adjusts to its new normal, it will easily adjust to the restrictions in calories, and you will be okay because the food that you will be eating will include nutrient-dense ingredients that will help your body feel satisfied.

Muscle Mass and Bones Preserved

Studies have shown that sirtuins can help boost muscle mass, especially in elderly individuals. If you want to make sure that your metabolism stays regulated, you must make sure that your muscles are there to help you, and if they are not, you can run into all sorts of problems. This means that if you really want to find a diet that will help you gain muscle and burn fat, the sirtuin rich Sirtfood Diet is one of the best for you.

Blood Sugar Levels under Control

Sirtuin-rich foods are known to inhibit the release of insulin improving blood sugar management. With the use of sirtuins, you are able to essentially prevent your blood sugar from dropping too low. This is a great point to keep in mind as compelling for completion of this diet, especially when you recognize that ultimately, you want to maintain that blood sugar so that you feel functional when restricting calories.

Improved Energy

Frequent meals help control blood sugar and hunger throughout the day, having a positive effect on energy level too thanks to sirtuins effect. As we will see later in the book, the Sirtfood Diet allows you to eat 5 times per day; juice, snack or meal depending on the phase of the diet you are in. Consumption of food with a low glycemic index may assist in the reduction of the lag in energy that occurs after taking food with fast absorption of sugars and refined starches.

Less Stress and Anxiety

Stress and large amounts of emotion consume a lot of energy in the body. Anxiety comes as a result of feeling anxious, sad, scared, or uncomfortable. Stress can be reduced in many forms, such as talking with friends or consulting with a psychotherapist. Sticking to regular mealtimes and planning meals can manage some of the stress.

Better Sleep

Sirtuin activators cause the SIR genes to activate, which in turn increases the release of SIRTs. SIRTs, or Silent Information Regulators also help regulate the circadian rhythm, which is your natural body clock and influences sleep patterns. Sleep is important for many vital biological processes, including those that help regulate blood sugar.

Anti-Aging Effect

Anti-aging is somehow linked to autophagy, which is an intracellular process of repairing or replacing damaged cell parts. This is rejuvenation occurs at an intracellular level. We can't mention autophagy without at least saying something about AMPK, an enzyme very important for cellular energy homeostasis. AMPK helps you boost the energy by activating fatty acid, glucose, and oxidation when the cellular energy is low. Well, SIRT1 can activate AMPK, so it can be considered one of the triggers of autophagy. Autophagy rejuvenates the cell, and this process can happen in all the cells of your body, from the ones of your internal organs to the ones of your skin.

Fights Chronic Diseases

As you already know, all bodies possess sirtuin genes, and activating them is crucial to burn fat and to build a stronger and leaner body. As it turns out, the benefits of sirtuins activity extend way beyond the fat-burning process. Whether we like it or not, the lack of sirtuins can be associated with plenty of diseases and medical conditions, while activating sirtuins will have the opposite effect. For example, sirtuins can play a major role in improving the function of your arteries, controlling the cholesterol level, and preventing atherosclerosis.

Cognitive Impairment and Alzheimer's

Individuals with Alzheimer's have been found to have notably lower levels of sirtuins than healthy peers, although the mechanism of action between sirtuin and the disease is not fully known. What is known is that the Sirtfood Diet helps prevent build-ups of amyloid-B and tau protein, molecules which are responsible for the plaques in the brains of people with Alzheimer's.

Diabetes

If you are suffering from diabetes, then you should know that activating sirtuins will make insulin work more effectively. Insulin is the hormone primarily responsible for controlling the levels of sugar in the blood. SIRT1 works perfectly with metformin.

Chapter 5

APPLICATION SIRTFOOD DIET PLANS

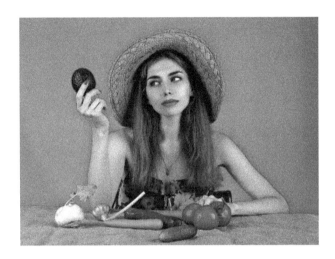

Eating some quality foods will improve the pathways of your "skinny gene" and allow you to shed some unnecessary weight in seven days. Food like kale, dark chocolate, and wine has a natural compound known as polyphenols that looks like fitness workout results and fasting. Strawberries, cinnamon and turmeric are also powerful sirt-foods. These foods can activate the steps or potentials of the sirtuin to help promote weight loss.

There are 2 phases to follow the sirtfood diet:

PHASE 1 Of The Sirtfood Diet

Calorie consumption is constrained to 1,000 calories in the initial three days (that is more than on a 5:2 day of fasting). The diet consists of 3 Sirtfood-full green juices and 1 Sirtfood-filled meal and 2 dark chocolate servings.

For the remaining 4 days calories intake should be raised to 1,500 calories and 2 sirtfood-filled green juices and 2 sirtfood-rich meals should be included daily in the diet.

You are not allowed to drink any alcohol in the early "Phase 1 stage," but you are free to take water and green tea.

PHASE 2 of the Sirtfood Diet

Phase 2 is not for reducing calorie consumption. Daily consumption includes 3 Sirtfood-rich foods and 1 green juice, and if possible the alternative of 1 or 2 Sirtfood crunch snacks.

You are permitted to take red wine in the second phase 2 but not too much (they encourage you to take 2-3 glasses of red wine weekly), as well as soda, tea, coffee and green tea too.

- PHASES OF THE SIRTFOOD DIET -

There are two phases for this diet; Phase 1 and Phase2

Phase 1: 7 pounds in seven days

MONDAY: three green juices

- Breakfast: water + tea or espresso + a cup of green juice;
- Lunch: green juice;
- Snack: a square of dark chocolate;
- Dinner: Sirt meal.
- After dinner: a square of dark chocolate.

Drink the juices at 3 different times of the day (for instance, in the morning as soon as you wake, mid-morning and mid-afternoon) and choose the usual or vegan dish: pan-fried oriental prawns with buckwheat spaghetti or miso and tofu with sesame glaze and sautéed vegetables (vegan dish).

TUESDAY: 3 green juices

- Breakfast: water + tea or espresso + a cup of green juice;
- Lunch: 2 green juices before dinner;
- Snack: a square of dark chocolate;
- Dinner: Sirt meal;
- After dinner: a square of dark chocolate.

Welcome to Sirtfood Diet day 2. The formula is similar to that of the first day, and only the solid meal varies. You'll have dark chocolate today, too, and the same will be true for tomorrow. This food is so amazing we don't need an excuse to eat it.

Chocolate must be at least 85% cocoa to receive the title of a "Sirt chocolate." And even with that percentage of the various types of chocolate, not all of them are the same. This substance is also treated with an alkalizing agent (the so-called "Netherlands process") to reduce its acidity and give it a darker color. Unfortunately this process greatly reduces the activation of sirtuins by flavonoids, compromising their health benefits. Lindt Excellence 85% chocolate, is not subject to the process in the Netherlands and is therefore often recommended.

The menu also includes capers on day 2, as well. They are not fruits, despite what many may think, but buds that grow in Mediterranean countries and are picked by hand. They are great Sirt foods, because they are very nutrient-rich

And quercetin and kaempferol. From the flavor standpoint, they are tiny taste concentrates. If you have never used them, feel no intimidation. You will see, if combined with the right ingredients, they will taste amazing, and will give your dishes an unmistakable and inimitable aroma.

You must consume on the second day: 3 green Sirt juices and one strong (normal or vegan) meal.

Drink the juices at three distinct times of the day (for example, when you wake up in the morning, mid-morning and mid-afternoon) and pick either the usual or vegan dish: turkey with capers, parsley and sage on spicy couscous or curly couscous cauliflower and buckwheat red onion Dahl (vegan dish).

———————————

WEDNESDAY: 3 green juices

- Breakfast: water + tea or espresso + a cup of green juice;
- Lunch: 2 green juices before dinner;
- Snack: a square of dark chocolate;
- Dinner: Sirt meal;
- After dinner: a square of dark chocolate.

You are now on the third day, and even though the style is again similar to that of days 1 and 2, then the time has come to spice it with a basic ingredient. Chili has been a fundamental element of the worldwide gastronomic experiences for thousands of years.

As for the health effects, we've already seen that its spiciness is perfect to activate sirtuins and stimulate metabolism. Chili's applications are endless, and thus provide a simple way to eat a daily Sirt meal.

If you're not a big chili expert, we recommend the Bird's Eye (sometimes called Thai chili), because, for sirtuins, it's the best.

This is the last day you consume three green juices a day; you switch to two tomorrow. And we take this opportunity to browse other beverages you may have during your diet. We all know that green tea is good for health and water is very good of course, but what about coffee? More than half of people drink at least one coffee a day, but still with a hint of shame because others claiming it's a crime and an unhealthy habit. Studies show that coffee is a true treasure trove of beneficial plant substances. That's why coffee drinkers are the least likely to get diabetes, certain forms of cancer, and neurodegenerative diseases. In addition, coffee isn't just a toxin, it protects the liver and makes it even healthier!

You will ingest 3 green Sirt juices and 1 solid meal on the third day (normal or vegan, see below).

Drink the juices at 3 different times of the day (e.g. in the morning as soon as you wake up, mid-morning and mid-afternoon) and pick the usual or vegan dish: aromatic chicken breast with kale, red onion, tomato sauce, and chili or baked tofu with harissa on spicy couscous (vegan platter).

THURSDAY: 2 green juices

- Breakfast: water + tea or espresso + a cup of green juice;
- Lunch: Sirt food;
- Snack: 1 green juice before dinner;
- Dinner: Sirt food.

The Sirtfood Diet's fourth day has arrived, and you are halfway through your journey into a leaner, healthier body. The big change from the previous three days is you're only going to drink two juices instead of three and you're going to have two solid meals in place of one. That means you'll have two green juices and two strong meals on the fourth day and the next day, all delicious and rich in Sirt foods. It may seem surprising to include Medjoul dates in a list of foods that support weight loss and good health. Especially if you think they have 66 percent sugar in them.

Sugar does not have any stimulating properties against sirtuins. On the contrary, it has well-known linkages with obesity, heart disease , and diabetes; in short, we target only at the antipodes of the targets. But industrially refined and processed sugar in a food which also contains sirtuin-activating polyphenols is very different from the sugar present: the Medjoul dates. These dates, consumed in moderation, do not increase blood glucose levels as opposed to normal sugar.

You must intake on the fourth day: 2 green Sirt juices, 2 solid meals (normal or vegan).

Drink the juices at various times of the day (for example the first in the morning as soon as you wake up or in the middle of the morning, the second in the middle of the afternoon) and select the normal or vegan dishes: muesli sirt, pan-fried salmon filet with caramelized chicory, rocket salad and celery leaves or muesli Sirt and Tuscan stewed beans (vegan dish).

FRIDAY: 2 green juices

- Breakfast: water + tea or espresso + a cup of green juice;
- Lunch: Sirt food;
- Snack: a green juice before dinner;
- Dinner: Sirt food.

You have hit the fifth day, so it's time to add some berries. Because of its high sugar content, fruit was the subject of bad advertisement. That is not applicable to berries. The sugar content of strawberries is very low: one teaspoon per 100 grams. They also have an excellent influence on how simple sugars are processed in the body.

Scientists have found that this causes a reduction in insulin demand if we add strawberries to simple sugars, and thus transforms food into a machine that releases energy for a long time to come. Therefore strawberries are a perfect diet element that will help you lose weight and get back into shape. They are also delicious and extremely versatile, as you'll discover the fresh and light Middle Eastern tabbouleh in the Sirt version.

The Miso is a popular Japanese soup, made from fermented soy. Miso has a powerful scent of umami, a complete explosion for the taste buds. We know better the monosodium glutamate in our modern society, produced artificially to replicate the same taste. Needless to say, deriving the magical umami taste from conventional and natural ingredients, full of beneficial substances, is much more preferable. It is found in all good supermarkets and healthy food stores in the form of a paste, and should be present in each kitchen to give many different dishes a touch of taste.

Because umami flavors enhance one another, miso is perfectly associated with other tasty / umami foods, particularly when it comes to cooked proteins, as you will discover in the very tasty, quick, and easy dishes you are going to eat today.

You will ingest 2 green Sirt juices and 2 solid (normal or vegan) meals on the fifth day.

Drink the juices at various times of the day (for instance; the first in the middle of the morning or as soon as you wake up; the second in the middle of the afternoon) and pick the usual or vegan dishes: buckwheat Tabbouleh with strawberries, baked cod marinated in miso with sautéed.

Sesame or buckwheat vegetables and strawberry Tabbouleh (vegan platter) and kale (vegan dish).

———————

SATURDAY: 2 green juices

- Breakfast: water + tea or espresso + a cup of green juice;
- Lunch: Sirt food;

- Snack: a green juice before dinner;
- Dinner: Sirt food.

There is no better Sirt food than the olive oil and red wine. Virgin olive oil is only obtained by mechanical means from the fruit, in conditions that do not deteriorate it, so you can be sure of its quality and polyphenol content. "Extra virgin" oil is the first pressing oil ("virgin" is the product of the second pressing) and thus has more flavor and higher quality: this is what we highly prefer to use while cooking.

No Sirt menu would be complete without red wine, which is one of the diet's cornerstones. It contains resveratrol and piceatannol sirtuins activators that are likely to explain the longevity and slenderness associated with the traditional French way of life and that are at the root of the enthusiasm unleashed by Sirt foods.

You'll expect 2 green Sirt juices and 2 strong (normal or vegan) meals on the sixth day.

Drink the juices at different times of the day (for example, the first in the middle of the morning or as soon as you wake up, the second in the middle of the afternoon) and choose the ordinary or vegan dishes: Super Sirt salad and grilled beef fillet with red wine sauce, onion rings, garlic curly kale and roasted potatoes with aromatic herbs, or Super lentil Sirt salad (vegan dish) and red bean mole sauce with roasted potato (vegan dish).

SUNDAY: 2 green juices

- Breakfast: a bowl of Sirt Muesli + a cup of green juice
- Lunch: Sirt food;
- Snack: a cup of green juice;
- Dinner: Sirt food.

The seventh day is the final of the diet's step 1. Instead of seeing it as an end, see it as a beginning, for you are about to embark on a new life in which sirt foods can play a central role in your diet. The today's menu is a perfect example of how easy it is to integrate them into your daily diet in abundance. Just take your favorite dishes, and turn them into a Sirt banquet with a pinch of imagination.

Walnuts are perfect Sirt food because they refute current views. They have a high-fat content and many calories, yet they have been shown to contribute to weight reduction and metabolic diseases, all thanks to sirtuin activation. Also, they are a versatile ingredient, excellent in baked dishes, salads, and alone as a snack.

We can apply the same reasoning to a dish which is easy to prepare, such as an omelet. The dish must be the traditional recipe that the whole family appreciates, and it must be easy to turn into a Sirt dish with a few little tricks. We use bacon in our recycle. Why? For what? Just because it just fits perfectly. The Sirtfood Diet tells us what to include, not what to exclude, and this allows us to change our eating habits over the long term. Isn't that, after all, the secret of not getting the lost pounds back and staying healthy?

You'll assume 2 green Sirt juices on the seventh day; 2 solid (normal or vegan) meals.

Drink the juices at different times of the day (for example the first in the morning as soon as you wake up or in the middle of the morning, the second in the middle of the afternoon) and choose the normal or vegan dishes: omelet sirt and boiled aubergine wedges with walnut and parsley pesto and tomato salad (vegan dish).

There are no calorie restrictions during the second phase but indications on which Sirt foods should be eaten to consolidate weight loss and not run the risk of getting the kilograms lost back.

Phase 2: Maintenance

Congratulations, you have finished the first "hard core" week. The second step is the simpler one and is the actual integration of food choices loaded with sirtuin into your daily diet or meals. You can call this the "stage of maintenance"

Your body will be subjected to the fat-burning level, and muscle gain plus a boost to your immune system and overall health.

You can now get 3 healthy SirtFood-filled meals per day for this process plus 1 green juice per day.

There is no "dieting" but more about selecting safer alternatives with as much as possible adding SirtFood to every meal. I will be providing some SirtFood inclusive recipes for tasty dishes to give you an idea of how exciting and healthy this diet journey is.

Now you are going back to a daily intake of calories with the intention of keeping your weight loss stable and your Sirtfood intake high. By now, you should have undergone a degree of weight loss, but you should still feel trimming and revitalizing.

Phase 2, which lasts 14 days. During this time you will eat 3 sirtfood-rich meals, 1 sirtfood-green juice and up to 2 optional snacks of Sirtfood bite. Strict calorie-counting is actively discouraged you follow recommendations and eat reasonable portions of balanced meals, you shouldn't feel hungry or consume too much.

You will have the same drinks you drank in step 1, with the small improvement you're welcome to enjoy the occasional glass of red wine (though you don't drink more than 3 a week).

Chapter 6
THE BEST 20 SIRTFOODS

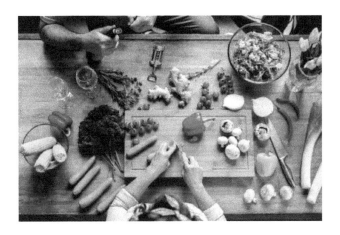

The list of the "top twenty sirtfoods" includes:

- **Arugula**
- **Buckwheat**
- **Capers**
- **Celery**
- **Chilies**
- **Cocoa**
- **Coffee**
- **Garlic**
- **Green Tea (Especially Matcha)**
- **Kale**
- **Medjool Dates**
- **Olive Oil (Extra Virgin)**
- **Parsley**
- **Red Endive**

- **Red Onions**
- **Red Wine**
- **Soy**
- **Strawberries**
- **Turmeric**
- **Walnuts**

The diet consolidates calorie and sirtfoods restriction, both of which may trigger the body to produce higher levels of sirtuins.

The developers of the diet say that following the Sirtfood diet would result in rapid weight loss, while retaining muscle mass and shielding you from chronic illness.

If you've finished the diet, you're allowed to continue your daily a diet including sirt foods and the signature green juice of the diet.

Arugula

Clearly, Arugula (also known as rocket, rucola, rugula, and roquette) has a colorful background in American food culture. A pungent green salad leaf with a distinctive peppery taste, it rapidly ascended from humble origins as the basis of many Mediterranean peasant dishes to become a symbol of food snobbery in the United States, also contributing to the coining of the word arugulance!

But long before it was a salad leaf wielded in a class war, arugula was revered by the ancient Greeks and Romans for its medicinal properties. Commonly used as a diuretic and digestive aid, it gained its true fame from its reputation for having potent aphrodisiac properties, so much so that growth of arugula was banned in monasteries in the Middle Ages, and the famous Roman poet Virgil wrote that "the rocket excites the sexual desire of drowsy people."

However, what really excites us about arugula is its bumper quantities of the sirtuin-activating kaempferol and quercetin nutrients. A combination of kaempferol and quercetin is being investigated as a cosmetic ingredient in addition to powerful sirtuin-activating properties because together they moisturize and enhance collagen synthesis in the skin. With those credentials, it's time to remove that elitist tag and make this the leaf of choice for salad bases, where it beautifully pairs with an extra virgin olive oil dressing, combining to create a strong double act of Sirtfood.

Buckwheat

Buckwheat was one of Japan's first domesticated crops, and the story goes that when Buddhist monks made long trips into the mountains, they'd only bring a cooking pot and a buckwheat bag for food. Buckwheat is so nutritious that this was all they wanted, and it kept them up for weeks. We're big fans of buckwheat too. Firstly, since it is one of a sirtuin activator's best-known outlets, named rutin. But also because it has advantages as a cover crop, improving soil quality and suppressing weed growth, making it a great crop for environmentally friendly and sustainable agriculture.

One reason buckwheat is head and shoulders above other, more popular grains is possible because it's not a grain at all — it's actually a rhubarb-related fruit seed. Having one of the highest protein content of any grain, as well as being a Sirtfood powerhouse, makes it an unrivaled alternative to more widely used grains. However, it is as flexible as any grain, and being naturally gluten-free, it is a perfect alternative for those intolerant to gluten.

Capers

In case you're not so familiar with capers, we're talking about those salty, dark green, pellet-like things on top of a pizza that you may only have had occasion to see. But certainly, they are one of the most undervalued and neglected foods out there. Intriguingly, they are actually the caper bush's flower buds, which grow abundantly in the Mediterranean before being picked and preserved by hand. Studies now show that capers possess important antimicrobial, antidiabetic, anti-inflammatory, immunomodulatory, and antiviral properties and have a rich history of being used as a medicine in the Mediterranean and North Africa. Hardly surprising when we discover that they are crammed full of sirtuin-activating nutrients.

We think it is about time these tiny morsels got their share of glory, too often overshadowed by the other big hitters from the Mediterranean diet. Flavor-wise it's a case of big stuff coming in small packages, as they're sure they're punching. Yet if you don't know how to use them then don't feel scared. For these diminutive nutrient superstars, when paired with the right ingredients have a wonderfully distinctive and inimitable sour / salty taste to round off a dish in style, we'll soon have you up to speed and falling head over heels.

Celery

For centuries, Celery was around and revered — with leaves found adorning the remains of the Egyptian pharaoh Tutankhamun who died around 1323 BCE. Early strains were very bitter, and celery was generally considered a medicinal plant for cleaning and detoxification to prevent disease. This is particularly interesting considering that liver, kidney, and gut safety are among the many promising benefits that science is now showing. It was domesticated as a vegetable in the seventeenth century, and selective breeding diminished its strong bitter flavor in favor of sweeter varieties, thus establishing its place as a traditional salad vegetable.

It is important to remember when it comes to celery, that there are two types: blanched / yellow and Pascal / green. Blanching is a technique developed to reduce the characteristic bitter taste of the celery, which has been considered to be too intense. It involves shading the celery before harvesting from sunshine, resulting in a paler color and a milder flavor. What a travesty that is, for blanching dumbs down the sirtuin-activating properties of celery as well as dumbing down the flavor. Thankfully, the tide is shifting and people are demanding true and distinct flavor, moving back to the greener variety. Green celery is the sort that we suggest you use in both the green juices and meals, with the heart and leaves being the most nutritious pieces.

Chilies

The chili has been an integral part of gastronomic experience worldwide for thousands of years. On one level it's disconcerting that we'd be so enamored with it. Its pungent fire, caused by a substance called capsaicin in chilies, is designed as a mechanism of plant defense to cause pain and dissuade predators from feasting on it, and we appreciate that. The food, and our infatuation with it, is almost mysterious.

Incredibly, one study found that consuming chilies together also enhances individual cooperation.[1] And we know from a health perspective that their seductive heat is great to stimulate our sirtuins and improve our metabolism. The culinary applications of the chili are also endless, making it a simple way to offer a hefty Sirtfood boost to any dish. While we understand that not everyone is a fan of hot or spicy food, we hope we can entice you to consider adding small amounts of chilies, particularly in light of recent studies showing that those consuming spicy foods three or more times a week have a 14 percent lower death risk compared to those consuming them less than once a week.

The hotter the chili, the stronger its Sirtfood credentials, but be careful and stick with what suits your own tastes. Serrano peppers are a great start-they are tolerable for most people when packing heat; and for more experienced heat seekers, we suggest looking for Thai chilies for optimum sirtuin-activating benefits. They can be difficult to find in grocery stores but are mostly sold in specialty markets in Asia. Opt for deep-colored peppers, avoiding those with a wrinkled and fuzzy appearance.

Cocoa

It's no surprise to learn that cocoa was considered a sacred food for ancient civilizations like the Aztecs and Mayans, and was usually reserved for the elite and warriors, served at feasts to gain loyalty and duty. Indeed, there was such high regard for the cocoa bean that it was even used as a form of currency. It was usually served as a frothy beverage back then. But what could be a more delicious way to get our dietary amount of cacao than by chocolate?

Unfortunately, there's no count here for the diluted, refined, and highly sweetened milk chocolate we commonly munch. We're talking about chocolate with 85 percent solids of cocoa to earn the Sirtfood badge. But even then, apart from the percentage of cocoa, not all chocolate is produced equal. To its acidity and give it a darker color, chocolate is often treated with an alkalizing agent (known as the Dutch process). Sadly, this process diminishes its sirtuin-activating flavanols significantly, thus seriously compromising its health-promoting content. Fortunately, and unlike in several other nations, food labeling laws in the United States allow alkalized cocoa to be reported as such and labeled "alkali processed." We suggest avoiding such items, even though they advertise a higher percentage of cocoa, and opting instead for those who have not undergone Dutch processing to enjoy the true benefits of cocoa.

Coffee

What's all that about Sirtfood Coffee? We're listening to you. We can assure you that this is no typo. Gone are the days when a twinge of remorse had to balance our enjoyment of coffee. The work is unambiguous: coffee is a bona fide food for wellbeing. Indeed it is a true treasure chest of fantastic nutrients that trigger sirtuin. And with more than half of Americans consuming coffee every day (to the tune of $40 billion a year!), coffee enjoys the accolade of becoming America's number one source of polyphenols.

The biggest irony is that the one thing we were chastised by so many fitness "experts" for doing was in reality the best thing we were doing for our wellbeing each day. This is why coffee drinkers have significantly less diabetes, and lower rates of some cancers and neurodegenerative disease. As for the ultimate irony, coffee, rather than being a poison, actually protects our livers and makes them healthier! And contrary to the common misconception that coffee dehydrates the body, it is now well known not to be the case, with coffee (and tea) contributing very well to daily coffee drinkers' fluid intake. And while we understand that coffee is not for everyone and some people might be very susceptible to the effects of caffeine, it's happy days for those who love a cup of joe.

Garlic

Garlic has been considered one of Nature's wonder foods for thousands of years, with soothing and rejuvenating properties. Egyptians fed pyramid workers with garlic to enhance their immunity, avoid various diseases, and strengthen their performance through their ability to resist fatigue. Garlic is a potent natural antibiotic and antifungal that is sometimes used to help cure ulcers in the stomach. By speeding the elimination of waste products from the body, it can stimulate the lymphatic system to "detox".

And as well as being investigated for fat loss, it also packs a potent heart health punch, lowering cholesterol by about 10 percent, and lowering blood pressure by 5 to 7 percent, as well as lowering blood stickiness and blood sugar levels.[7] And if you're worried about the off-putting garlic odor, note. When women were asked to assess a selection of men's body odors, those men who ingested four or more garlic cloves a day were found to have a much more attractive and friendly odor. Researchers suggest this is because it is viewed as signaling better health. And there's always mints for fresher breath of course!

Eating garlic has a trick to get full profit. In garlic, the Sirtfood nutrients are complemented by another key nutrient in it called allicin, which gives off the characteristic aroma of garlic. But after physical "injury" to the bulb allicin only forms in garlic. And, when exposed to heat (cooking) or low pH (stomach acid), its formation is halted. So when preparing garlic, chop, thin, or crush, and then allow it to sit for about ten minutes before cooking or eating the allicin.

Green Tea (Especially Matcha)

Many will be familiar with green tea, the toast of the Orient and ever more popular in the West. With the rising awareness of its health benefits, green tea consumption is related to less cancer , heart disease, diabetes and osteoporosis. The reason it is thought that green tea is so good for us is primarily due to its rich content of a group of powerful plant compounds called catechins, the star of the show being a particular type of sirtuin-activating catechin known as epigallocatechin gallate (EGCG).

But what the fuss about matcha is all about? We like to think of matcha on the steroids as normal green tea. In comparison to traditional green tea, which is prepared as an infusion, it is a special powdered green tea which is prepared by dissolving directly in water. The upshot of drinking matcha is that it contains significantly higher levels of the sirtuin-activating compound EGCG than other green tea forms. Zen priests describe matcha as the "ultimate mental and medical remedy [which] has the potential to make one 's life more full" if you are looking for more endorsement.

Kale

We are at heart cynics, so we are always skeptical about what drives the latest craze for superfood advertising. Was it science, or is it interests at stake? In recent years few foods have exploded as dramatically as kale on the health scene. Described as the "lean, green brassica queen" (referring to its cruciferous vegetable family), it has become the chic vegetable for which all health-lovers and foodies are gunning. Every October there is also a National Day of the Kale. But you don't have to wait until then to show your kale pride: there are T-shirts too, with trendy slogans such as "Powered by Kale" and "Highway to Kale." That's enough for us to set the alarm bells ringing. We've done the research, filled with suspicions, and we have to admit that our conclusion is that kale really deserves her pleasures (although we still don't recommend the T-shirts!). The reason we're pro-kale is that it boasts bumper quantities of the quercetin and kaempferol sirtuin-activating nutrients, making it a must-include in the Sirtfood Diet and the foundation of our green Sirtfood juice. What's so exciting about kale is that kale is available anywhere, locally produced, and very inexpensive, unlike the typical expensive, hard-to-source, and exorbitantly priced so-called superfoods!

Medjool Dates

It that comes as a surprise to include Medjool dates in a list of foods that stimulate weight loss and promote health—especially when we tell you that Medjool dates contain a staggering 66 percent sugar. Sugar doesn't have any sirtuin-activating properties at all; rather, it has well-established links to obesity, heart disease, and diabetes — just the opposite of what we're looking to achieve. Yet processed and refined sugar is very different from sugar borne in a naturally supplied vehicle filled with sirtuin-activating polyphenols: the date of the Medjool.

Medjool dates, consumed in moderation, do not really have any real significant blood-sugar-raising effects, in complete contrast with regular sugar. Instead, eating them is associated with developing less diabetes and heart disease. They have been a staple food worldwide for centuries, and there has been an explosion of scientific interest in dates in recent years, which sees them emerging as a potential medicine for a number of diseases. Herein lies the uniqueness and power of the Sirtfood Diet: it refutes the dogma and allows you to indulge in sweet things in moderation without feeling guilty.

Olive Oil (Extra Virgin)

Olive oil is the most renowned of Mediterranean traditional diets. The olive tree is among the world's oldest-known cultivated plants, also known as the "immortal tree." And since people started squeezing olives in stone mortars to gather them, the oil has been respected, almost 7,000 years ago. Hippocrates cited it as a cure-all; now, a few decades later, modern science confidently claims its wonderful health benefits.

There is now a wealth of scientific information showing that regular olive oil consumption is highly cardioprotective, as well as playing a role in reducing the risk of major modern-day diseases such as diabetes, certain cancers, and osteoporosis, and associated with increased longevity.

Parsley

Parsley is a food conundrum. It appears so often in recipes, and so often it's the token green man. At best we serve a couple of chopped sprigs and tossed as an afterthought on a meal, at worst a single sprig for decorative purposes only. That way, there on the plate it is always languishing long after we have finished eating. This culinary style stems from its common use in ancient Rome as a garnish for eating after meals to refresh breath, rather than being part of the meal itself. And what a shame, because parsley is a wonderful food that packs a vivid, refreshing taste full of character.

Taste aside, what makes parsley very unique is that it is an excellent source of the sirtuin-activating nutrient apigenin, a real blessing because it is rarely contained in other foods in large amounts. In our brains, apigenin binds fascinatingly to the benzodiazepine receptors, helping us to relax and help us to sleep. Stack it all up, and it's time we appreciated parsley not as omnipresent food confetti, but as a food in its own right to reap the wonderful health benefits that it can offer.

Red Endive

Endive is a fairly new kid on the block in so far as vegetables go. Legend has it that a Belgian farmer found endive in 1830, by mistake. The farmer stored chicory roots in his cellar, and then used them as a type of coffee substitute, only to forget them. Upon his return, he discovered that white leaves had sprouted, which he found to be tender, crunchy, and rather delicious upon degustation.

Endive is now grown all over the world, including the USA, and earns its Sirtfood badge thanks to its impressive sirtuin activator luteolin content. And besides the proven sirtuin-activating benefits, luteolin intake has become a promising approach to therapy to enhance sociability in autistic children.

It has a sweet taset and crisp texture for those new to endive, followed by a gentle and friendly bitterness. If you're ever stuck on how to increase endive in your diet, you can't fail by adding her leaves to a salad where her warm, tart flavor adds the perfect bite to an extra virgin olive oil dressing based on zesty. Red is best, just like onion, but the yellow variety can also be considered a Sirtfood. So while the red variety may sometimes be more difficult to find, you can rest assured that yellow is a perfectly appropriate alternative.

Red Onions

Since the time of our prehistoric predecessors, onions have been a dietary staple, being one of the earliest crops to be cultivated, some 5,000 years ago. With such a long history of use and such potent health-giving properties, many cultures that came before us have revered onions. They were held especially by the Egyptians as objects of worship, regarding their circle-within-a-circle structure as symbolic of eternal life.

And the Greeks claimed that onions made athletes stronger. Athletes will eat their way through large quantities of oignons before the Olympic Games, even drinking the water! It's an amazing testament to how important ancient culinary knowledge can be when we remember that onions deserve their top twenty Sirtfood status because they're chock-full of the sirtuin-activating compound quercetin — the very compound that the sports science community has recently started aggressively researching and promoting to boost sports performance.

And why the red ones? Simply because they have the highest content of quercetin, although the regular yellow ones do not lag too far behind, and are also a good inclusion.

Red Wine

Any list of the top twenty Sirtfoods will not be complete without the inclusion of the original Sirtfood, red wine. The French phenomenon made headlines in the early 1990s, with it being discovered that despite the French appearing to do something wrong when it came to health (smoking, lack of exercise, and rich food consumption), they had lower death rates from heart disease than countries like the United States. The explanation for this was suggested by doctors was the copious amount of red wine drank. Danish researchers then published work in 1995 to show that low-to-moderate consumption of red wine decreased death rates, while comparable levels of beer alcohol had no effect, and comparable intakes of hard liquors increased death rates. Obviously, in 2003, the rich quality of red wine from a bevy of sirtuin-activating nutrients was discovered, and the rest, as they claim, was made history.

But there is much more to the outstanding resume of red wine. Red wine seems to be able to stop the common cold, with moderate wine drinkers seeing a reduction in its incidence of more than 40%. Studies also show benefits for oral health and cavity prevention. With moderate consumption, social interaction and out-of-the-box thinking have also been shown to increase the after-work drink between cavities.

It appears that colleagues debating work ventures have roots in solid research.

Moderation is of course important. To gain from this, only small quantities are required and excess alcohol quickly undoes the good. The sweet spot seems to stick up to one 5-ounce drink per day for women and up to two 5-ounce drinks per day for men according to US guidelines. Wines from the New York region (especially pinot noir, cabernet sauvignon, and merlot) have the highest polyphenol content of the most widely available wines to ensure maximum sirtuin-activating bang for your buck.

Soy

Soy products have a long history as an integral part of the diet of many countries in Asia-Pacific such as China, Japan, and Korea. Researchers first turned on to soy after discovering that high soy-consuming countries had significantly lower rates of certain cancers, especially prostate and breast cancers. It is believed to be attributed to a specific category of polyphenols in soybeans known as isoflavones, which can favorably affect how estrogens function in the body, like daidzein and formononetin sirtuin-activators. Soy product intake has also been related to a decrease in the incidence or severity of a number of conditions such as effects of menopause, cardiovascular disease, and bone loss.

Highly refined, nutrient-stripped soybean types are now a common component applied to various packaged foods. The benefits are only reaped from natural soy products such as tofu, an excellent vegan protein source, or in a fermented form such as tempeh, natto, or our favorite, miso, a typical Japanese paste fermented with a naturally occurring fungus that results in an intense umami taste.

Strawberries

In recent years, the fruit has been particularly vilified, getting a bad rap in the rising fervor toward sugar. Fortunately, such a malignant image couldn't be more undeserved for berry-lovers. While all berries are powerhouses of nutrition, strawberries are earning their top twenty Sirtfood status due to their abundance of the fisetin sirtuin activator. And now studies endorse daily eating strawberries to encourage healthy aging, keeping off Alzheimer's, cancer, diabetes, heart disease, and osteoporosis. It's very small as to their sugar content, a pure teaspoon of sugar per 3 / ounces.

Amusingly, and naturally low in sugar itself, strawberries have marked effects on how the body treats carbohydrates. What researchers have found is that adding strawberries to carbohydrates decreases the need for insulin, effectively transforming the food into a constant energy releaser. Yet recent work also shows that eating strawberries in diabetes treatment has close results to the drug therapy. William Butler, the great physician of the seventeenth century, wrote in praise of the strawberry: " God might have made a better berry, however, without doubt, He never did." We can only agree.

Turmeric

Turmeric, a cousin of ginger, is the new kid in food trends on the block, with Google naming it the ingredient of the 2015 breakout star. While we are only turning to it nowhere in the West, it has been valued for thousands of years in Asia, for both culinary and medical reasons. Incredibly, India is generating almost the entire world's turmeric supply, consuming 80% of it itself. In Asia, turmeric is used for treating skin disorders such as acne, psoriasis, dermatitis, and rash. Before Indian weddings, there is a ritual where the turmeric paste is applied as a skin beauty treatment to the bride and groom but also to symbolize the warding off evil.

One factor that limits turmeric's effectiveness is that the main sirtuin-activating compound, curcumin, is poorly absorbed by the body as we consume it. Analysis, however, shows that we can solve this by boiling it in oil, adding fat, and adding black pepper, all of which increase its absorption dramatically.

This suits well with traditional Indian cuisine, wherein curries and other hot dishes it is traditionally mixed with ghee and black pepper, and again prove that science just catches up with the age-old wisdom of traditional eating methods.

Walnuts

Dating back to 7000 BCE, walnuts are the oldest known tree food, originating in ancient Persia, where they were the preserve of royalty. Fast-forward to today and walnuts are a success story for the United States. California is leading the way, with California's Central Valley famous for being the prime walnut-growing area. California walnuts provide the United States with 99% of commercial supply and whopping three-quarters of worldwide walnut trade.

Walnuts lead the way as the number one nut for health, according to the NuVal system which ranks foods according to how safe they are and has been endorsed by the American College of Preventive Medicine. But what really makes walnuts stand out for us is how they fly in the face of traditional thinking: they are high in fat and calories, but well-established for weight loss and the risk of metabolic diseases like cardiovascular disease and diabetes is reduced. That is the strength of triggering the sirtuin.

The recent research showing walnuts to be an effective anti-aging food is less well known but equally fascinating. Research also points to their benefits as a brain food with the potential to slow down brain aging and reduce the risk of degenerative brain disorders, as well as preventing the decline in physical function with age.

Chapter 7

THE PERFECT SIRTFOOD RECIPES FOR ALL MEALS

BREAKFAST

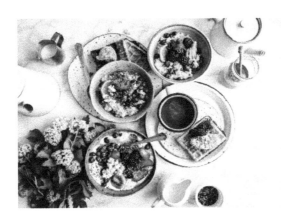

SIRT CEREAL

Ingredients

- Buckwheat, 1 oz flakes, and 0.5 oz puffs
- Coconut, either desiccated or flakes, 1.5 oz
- Chopped walnuts, 1.5 oz
- Medjool dates, 1.5 oz
- Chopped strawberries, 3.5 oz
- Cocoa nibs 0.5 oz
- Skim milk, almond/coconut milk or Greek yogurt, plain, 3.5 oz

Directions

Soak the dry ingredients in yogurt or milk and top with chopped strawberries. This meal is simple, delicious, and satiating. If you won't be eating right away, serve the yogurt and strawberries las.

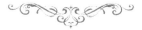

BUCKWHEAT WITH NUTS AND COCONUT

Ingredients

- Soy, coconut, or Greek yogurt, 100 g
- Walnuts, chopped, 0. 5 oz
- Buckwheat flakes, ½ cup
- Buckwheat puffs, ⅓ cup
- Coconut flakes or dried coconut, 0. 5 oz
- Chopped Medjool dates, 1.5 oz
- Cocoa nibs, 1.4 oz
- Chopped strawberries, 1 cup

Directions

Mix all ingredients and enjoy! If you want to have this mixture ready beforehand, you can mix the dry ingredients and store them in a container. Add yogurt only when you're about to serve.

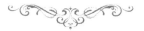

PANCAKES WITH BLUEBERRIES, BANANA AND APPLES

Ingredients

- For Pancakes
- Six bananas
- Blueberries, ¼ cup

- Six eggs
- Rolled oats, 1 ½ cup
- A pinch of salt
- Baking powder, 2 tsp
- For the applesauce
- Two apples
- Two pitted dates
- Lemon juice, 1 tbsp
- A pinch of cinnamon powder
- A pinch of salt
- For Turmeric Topping
- Coconut milk, 3 cup
- Ginger root, 1 small piece
- Raw honey, 1 tsp
- Turmeric powder, 1 tsp

Directions

Start by making your pancakes. First, make the oat flower by pulling the rolled oats in your blender for a minute. Add the remaining ingredients for the batter and blend for two minutes until you've formed a smooth batter. Pour the batter into a bowl and mix in blueberries, making sure that they are evenly distributed across the mixture.

Leave to sit for another 10 minutes until the baking powder is activated. Bake on medium on a thin layer of butter or coconut oil. To fry the pancakes evenly, distribute a couple of batter spoons across the pan, wait until it turns golden color, and flip to the other side.

Once your pancakes are done, start making the sauce. This step should be simple, and it consists of putting all the ingredients for the sauce into a blender and blending until the mixture is uniform.

Now, onto the turmeric topping. Pop all the ingredients into a blender, and then transfer into a small pot and heat on low temperature. The ingredients should melt together to form a syrup-like consistency, but not boil to avoid destroying the nutrients.

LEMONY MINT PANCAKES WITH YOGURT SAUCE

Ingredients

For The Yogurt Sauce
- One cup plain Greek yogurt
- One garlic clove, minced
- One to Two tablespoons lemon juice (from 1 lemon), to taste
- ¼ teaspoon ground turmeric
- Ten fresh mint leaves, minced
- Two teaspoons lemon zest (from 1 lemon)

For The Pancakes
- Two teaspoons ground turmeric
- 1½ teaspoons ground cumin
- One teaspoon salt
- 1 teaspoon ground coriander
- ½ teaspoon garlic powder
- ½ teaspoon freshly ground black pepper
- One head broccoli, cut into florets
- 3 large eggs, lightly beaten
- 2 tablespoons plain unsweetened almond milk
- Four teaspoons coconut oil
- One cup almond flour

Directions

1. Make the yogurt sauce. Mix the yogurt, turmeric, mint, zest, garlic, and lemon juice in a bowl. Taste and season with more lemon juice. Refrigerate until ready to serve.
2. Make the pancakes. combine the turmeric, coriander, garlic, cumin, salt, and pepper in a small bowl.
3. Put the broccoli in a food processor, and pulse until florets are broken up into pieces. Move the broccoli to a large bowl and add the milk, almond flour, eggs, and almond. Stir and combine well.

4. Heat one teaspoon of coconut oil over medium-low heat in a nonstick pan. Pour ¼ cup of batter into the skillet. Cook the pancake until the top starts to show tiny bubbles and the bottom is golden brown. Flip the pancake over and cook it for another 2 to 3 minutes. Switch the cooked pancakes to an oven-safe dish to keep warm, and put them in a 200 ° F oven.
5. Keep making the remaining three pancakes, using the remaining butter and oil.

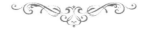

CHOCOLATE GRANOLA

Planning time: 60 Min. / Cooking time: 50 Min. / Servings: 2

Ingredients

- Four cups old-fashioned oats*
- One cup slivered almonds (or your preferred nuts)
- 1/3 cup unsweetened cocoa powder
- One teaspoon fine sea salt
- 1/2 cup melted coconut oil
- 1/2 cup maple syrup
- Two teaspoons vanilla extract
- 1/2 cup semisweet chocolate chips (optional)
- 1/2 cup shredded coconut (or 2/3 cup unsweetened flaked coconut)

Instructions

1. Heat the oven to 350 degrees. Line a large baking sheet and set it aside with parchment paper.
2. Stir the oats, almonds, cocoa powder, and sea salt together in a large bowl and mix until evenly mixed.
3. Stir together the melted coconut oil, vanilla extract, and maple syrup in a separate mixing cup, until mixed. Pour the coconut oil mixture into the oats mixture and whisk until evenly mixed.

4. On the prepared baking sheet, spread the granola out evenly. Bake, stirring once halfway through, for twenty minutes. Then remove it from the oven, add a good stir to the mixture, then sprinkle the coconut on top evenly. Bake until the granola is lightly toasted and golden.

5. Remove and transfer the baking sheet from the oven to a wire baking rack. Let the granola cool until it reaches room temperature. Then stir in the chocolate chips or/and any other add-ins.

6. Serve immediately, or place it in an airtight jar for up to 1 month at room temperature.

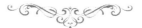

SIRTFOOD MELON SMOOTHIE

Ingredient

- ¼ cantaloupe - peeled, seeded, and cubed
- ¼ honeydew melon - peeled, seeded, and cubed
- 1 lime, juiced
- 2 tablespoons sugar

Directions

In a blender, combine cantaloupe, honeydew, lime juice, and sugar. Blend until smooth. Pour into glasses and serve.

Nutrition Facts: Per Serving: 70 calories; protein 0.8g 2% DV; carbohydrates 18.1g 6% DV; fat 0.2g; cholesterol mg; sodium 20.3 mg 1% DV.

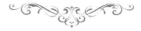

SIRTFOOD SMOOTHIE

Ingredient

- Berries of your choosing, 2 cup
- 1 ripe banana
- Greek yogurt, 2 tbsp

- Skim milk, 200 ml

Directions

Blend all the ingredients together and enjoy!

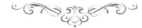

PREPARED PAN WITH CASHEW NUTS

Planning time: 30 min. / Cooking time: 0 min. / Servings: 2

Ingredients

- 150 g Pak choi
- 2 tablespoons Coconut oil 2 pieces Red onion
- 2 pieces yellow chime pepper 250 g White cabbage
- 50 g Mung bean grows 4 pieces Pineapple cuts 50 g Cashew nuts
- For the prepared sauce:
- 60 ml Apple juice vinegar
- 1 teaspoon Coconut-Aminos 2 teaspoon Arrowroot powder 75 ml Water
- 4 tablespoon Coconut bloom sugar 1½ tablespoon Tomato paste

Directions

1. Generally cut the vegetables.
2. Blend the bolt root with five tablespoons of cold water into a paste.
3. At that point put the various elements for the sauce in a pan and include the arrowroot paste for official.
4. Melt the coconut oil in a container and fry the onion.
5. Include the ringer pepper, cabbage, pak choi and bean sprouts and sautéed food until the vegetables become somewhat milder.
6. Include the pineapple and cashew nuts and mix a couple of more occasions.
7. Pour a little sauce over the wok dish and serve.

Nourishment: Calories: 573 kcal Protein: 15.25 g Fat: 27.81 g Starches: 77.91 g

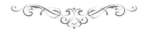

MOROCCAN SPICED EGGS

Planning time: 60 min. / Cooking time: 50 min. / Servings: 2

Ingredients:

- 1 tsp olive oil
- One shallot, stripped and finely hacked
- One red (chime) pepper, deseeded and finely hacked
- One garlic clove, stripped and finely hacked
- One courgette (zucchini), stripped and finely hacked
- 1 tbsp tomato puree (glue)
- ½ tsp gentle stew powder
- ¼ tsp ground cinnamon
- ¼ tsp ground cumin
- ½ tsp salt
- One × 400g (14oz) can hacked tomatoes
- 1 x 400g (14oz) may chickpeas in water
- a little bunch of level leaf parsley (10g (1/3oz)), cleaved
- Four medium eggs at room temperature

Directions:

1. Heat the oil in a pan, include the shallot and red (ringer) pepper and fry delicately for 5 minutes. At that point include the garlic and courgette (zucchini) and cook for one more moment or two. Include the tomato puree (glue), flavours and salt and mix through.
2. Add the cleaved tomatoes and chickpeas (dousing alcohol and all) and increment the
3. warmth to medium. With the top of the dish, stew the sauce for 30 minutes - ensure it is delicately rising all through and permit it to lessen in volume by around 33%.
4. Remove from the warmth and mix in the cleaved parsley.
5. Preheat the grill to 200C/180C fan/350F.
6. When you are prepared to cook the eggs, bring the tomato sauce up to a delicate stew and move to a little broiler confirmation dish.
7. Crack the eggs on the dish and lower them delicately into the stew. Spread with thwart and prepare in the grill for 10-15 minutes. Serve the blend in unique dishes with the eggs coasting on the top.

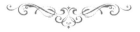

SALAD

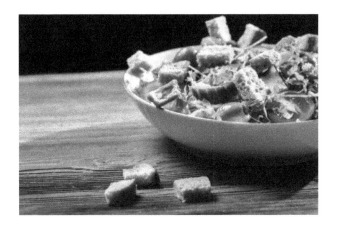

SIRTFOOD VEGETABLE SALAD

Ingredients

- 1 finely chopped apple
- Chopped celery, 200 g
- One roughly chopped red onion
- Roughly chopped walnuts, ½ cup
- 1 chopped chicory head
- Chopped parsley, 10 g
- Arugula, 1 tbsp
- Roughly chopped celery leaves,
- Extra virgin olive oil, 1 tbsp
- Lemon juice, ½ tbsp
- Mustard, 1 tsp

Directions

Mix the celery, arugula, onion, walnuts, and parsley in a bowl and toss together. Mix the extra virgin olive oil, lemon juice, and mustard. Drizzle over the salad and enjoy!

QUINOA AND AVOCADO SALAD

Planning time: 10 Min. / Cooking Time: 20 Min./ Servings 4

Ingredients

- 1 cup quinoa
- 2 cups water
- 1 large avocado, pitted and sliced
- ¼ radicchio, finely sliced
- 1 small pink grapefruit, peeled and finely cut
- 1 handful arugula
- 1 cup baby spinach leaves
- 2 tbsp extra virgin olive oil
- 2 tbsp lemon juice
- Salt and black pepper, to taste

Directions

Wash quinoa in a fine sieve under running water for 3-4 minutes, or until water runs clear. Set aside to drain, then boil it in two cups of water for 16 minutes.

Fluff with a fork and set aside to cool. Stir avocado, radicchio, arugula and baby spinach into cooled quinoa.

Add grapefruit, lemon juice, and olive oil, season with salt and black pepper and stir to combine well.

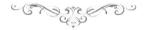

CARROT, BUCKWHEAT, TOMATO AND ARUGULA SALAD IN A JAR

Planning time: 5 Min. / Cooking Time: 30 Min./ Servings 2

Ingredients

- 1/2 cup sunflower seeds 1/2 cup carrots
- 1/2 cup of tomatoes
- 1 cup cooked buckwheat blended in with 1 tbsp.
- chia seeds 1 cup arugula
- 1/2 cup of destroyed cabbage
- Dressing:
- 1 tbsp. olive oil
- 1 tbsp. new lemon juice and place of ocean salt

Directions

1. Put ingredients in a specific order: dressing, sunflower seeds, carrots, cabbage, tomatoes, buckwheat, and arugula.

Nourishment: Calories: 293 kcal Protein: 8.46 g Fat: 25.02 g Starches: 13.62 g

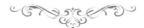

CUCUMBER SALAD WITH LIME AND CORIANDER

Ingredients

- 1 piece Red onion 2 pieces Cucumber
- 2 tablespoons new coriander
- 2 pieces Lime (juice)

Directions

8. Cut the onion into rings and daintily cut the cucumber. Slice the coriander finely.
9. Place the onion rings in a bowl and season with about a large portion of a tablespoon of salt. Focus on it well and afterward fill the bowl with water.
10. Pour off the water and afterward flush the onion rings completely (in a strainer).

11. Set up the cucumber cuts with onion, lime juice, coriander, and olive oil in a salad bowl and mix everything great.
12. Season with somewhat salt.
13. You can keep this dish in the cooler in a secured bowl for a couple of days.
Nourishment: Calories: 57 kcal Protein: 2 g Fat: 0.41 g Starches: 13.22 g

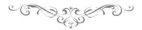

CHICKPEAS, ONION, TOMATO AND PARSLEY SALAD IN A JAR

Planning time: 5 Min. / Cooking Time: 50 Min. / Servings 2

Ingredients

- 1/2 of a little onion, sliced 1 tbsp. chia seeds
- 1 Tbsp. sliced parsley
- 1 cup cooked chickpeas 1/2 cup sliced tomatoes

Dressing:

- 1 tbsp. olive oil and 1 tbsp. of Chlorella.
- 1 tbsp. new lemon juice and a touch of ocean salt

Directions

1. Put ingredients in a specific order: dressing, tomatoes, chickpeas, onions, and parsley.
Nourishment: Calories: 210 kcal Protein: 7.87 g Fat: 9 g Starches: 26.22 g

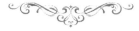

KALE AND FETA SALAD WITH CRANBERRY DRESSING

Planning time: 5 Min. / Cooking Time: 30 Min. / Servings 2

Ingredients

- 9oz kale, finely sliced 2oz walnuts, cleaved 3oz feta cheese, disintegrated
- 1 apple, stripped, cored and cut
- 4 Medjool dates, sliced
- For the Dressing 3oz cranberries
- ½ red onion, sliced 3 tablespoons olive oil 3 tablespoons water
- 2 teaspoons nectar
- 1 tablespoon red wine vinegar Sea salt.

Directions

1. Place the elements for the dressing into a food processor and procedure until smooth. If it appears to be too thick you can include some additional water if important. Place all the elements for the salad into a bowl. Pour on the dressing and hurl the salad until it is all around covered in the blend.

Nourishment: Calories: 706 kcal Protein: 15.62 g Fat: 45.92 g Starches: 70.28 g

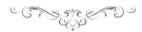

ARUGULA SALAD

Ingredients

- 2 tablespoons olive oil
- 2 tablespoons
- freshly squeezed lemon juice
- 1/8 teaspoon kosher salt
- Freshly ground black pepper
- 5 ounces arugula (about 5 packed cups)
- 2 ounces shaved Parmesan cheese (about 2/3 cup)

Directions

1. Whisk the lemon juice, olive oil, salt, and a few grinds of black pepper together in a large bowl. Add the arugula and toss to combine. Top with the shaved Parmesan and serve immediately.

APPLE AND LIME SIRTFOOD SALAD

Ingredients

- 1 green apple
- 6 chopped walnuts
- Chopped celery, 1 cup
- Finely chopped ginger, 1 tbsp
- Chopped Kale, 1 cup
- Lime juice, 1 tbsp
- Parsley, 1 tbsp
- Arugula, 1 cup
- A pinch of salt
- A pinch of pepper
- Extra virgin olive oil, 1 tbsp

Directions

Mix all of the ingredients together and enjoy!

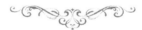

QUICK SIRTFOOD CHICKEN SALAD

Ingredients

- Diced chicken breasts, 5 oz
- Greek yogurt, 1 cup
- Lime juice, 1 tbsp
- Ground turmeric, 1 tsp
- Chopped coriander, 1 tsp
- Curry powder, ½ tsp
- Chopped walnuts, 1 cup
- 2 finely chopped Medjool dates
- Arugula, 1 cup

- 1 bird's eye chili
- 1 diced red onion

Directions

1. Cook chicken breasts until ready per your taste and set aside to cool down.
2. Mix the dry ingredients into a bowl, add the chicken breasts, top with lime juice and extra virgin olive oil.

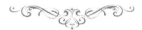

BRAISED LEEK WITH PINE NUTS

Planning time: 45 minutes / Cooking time 15 min / Servings 2

Ingredients

- 20 g Ghee
- 1 tablespoon new oregano
- tablespoon Pine nuts (simmered)
- 2 teaspoon Olive oil 2 pieces Leek
- 150 ml Vegetable stock new parsley ....

Directions

1. Cut the leek into thin rings and finely slice the herbs. Cook the pine nuts in a dry pan over medium warmth.
2. Melt the ghee along with the olive oil in a huge pan.
3. Cook the leek until brilliant brown for 5 minutes, blending continually.
4. Include the vegetable stock and cook for an additional 10 minutes until the leek is delicate. Mix in the herbs and sprinkle the pine nuts on the dish not long before serving.

Nutrition: Calories: 95 kcal Protein: 1.35 g Fat: 4.84 g Sugars: 12.61 g.

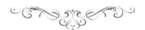

FISH, EGG AND CAPER SALAD

Planning time: 5 Min. / Cooking Time: 20 Min. / Servings 2

Ingredients

- 1 tablespoon escapades
- 2 tablespoons garlic vinaigrette
- 2 hard-boiled eggs, stripped and quartered
- 3½ozred chicory or yellow if not accessible 5oz tinned fish drops in saline solution, depleted
- 3 ½ oz cucumber 1oz rocket arugula 6 pitted dark olives
- 2 tomatoes, cut
- 2 tablespoons new parsley, cut 1 red onion, sliced
- 1 stem of celery

Directions

1. Place the fish, cucumber, olives, tomatoes, onion, chicory, celery, parsley and rocket arugula into a bowl. Pour in the vinaigrette and prepare the salad in the dressing. Serve onto plates and disperse the eggs and escapades on top.

Nutrition: Calories: 309 kcal Protein: 26.72 g Fat: 12.23 g Sugars: 25.76 g

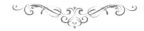

BUCKWHEAT AND STRAWBERRIES SALAD

Planning time: 10 Min. / Cooking Time: 3 Min. / Servings 2

Ingredients

- 50 g buckwheat
- 1 tbsp. ground Tumeric
- 80 g avocado
- 65 g tomato
- 20 g red onion
- 25 g Medjool dates, pitted
- 1 tbsp. capers
- 30 g parsley

- 100 g strawberries, hulled
- 1 tbsp. extra virgin olive oil
- juice of 1/2 lemon
- 30 g rocket

Directions

Cook the buckwheat with the turmeric according to the packet directions. Drain and keep to one side to cool.

Chop the tomato, red onion, avocado, dates, parsley, and capers and mix with the cool buckwheat. Slice the strawberries and gently blend the oil and lemon juice into the salad. Serve on a bed of rocket.

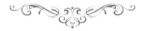

MISO AND SESAME GLAZED TOFU WITH GINGER AND CHILI STIR-FRIED GREENS

Prep time: 15 Min. / Cooking time: 25 Min. / Serves: 2

Ingredients

- Two tablespoon mirin
- Two tablespoons (40g) brown miso paste
- 250g firm tofu
- One stick of celery, trimmed, stringy pieces peeled away and chopped finely
- One red onion, sliced thin
- One courgette, sliced thin
- Two bird's eye chili, seeds removed and finely chopped (optional as quite spicy)
- Two garlic cloves, finely chopped
- Two teaspoons fresh ginger, finely chopped
- Four teaspoon sesame seeds
- 100g (1 1/4 cup) kale, washed and chopped
- 235 ml (1 cup) water
- 70g (1/2cup) buckwheat or buckwheat noodles
- Two teaspoon ground turmeric
- Four teaspoons extra virgin olive oil

- Two teaspoon tamari

Directions

1. Preheat your oven to 200°C/gas 6
2. Line a small roasting tin with parchment or greaseproof paper.
3. Mix the miso and mirin together in a bowl. Cut the tofu, then cut each piece in half, forming triangles. With the miso mixture, cover the tofu and leave to marinate as you are preparing the other ingredients.
4. Cook the kale in a steamer for five minutes, remove it and leave it on one side. Place a pan of water on the hob and bring to a rolling boil; place a collider over the top of the kale; this will serve as a steamer if you don't have one.
5. Slice the trimmed celery, red onion, and courgette in the corner while the kale is cooking. Then the chili (making sure all seeds are removed), garlic, and ginger are thinly chopped and left on one side.
6. In the roasting pan, put the marinated tofu, sprinkle the sesame seeds over the tofu, and roast for twenty minutes until nicely caramelized.
7. Wash the buckwheat in a sieve and boil a cup of water, adding the turmeric and a pinch of salt to taste. Attach the buckwheat and leave it on high heat until the water has started boiling. When buckwheat has expanded and started to absorb the water, reduce to low heat, and put the lid on, cook for fifteen minutes. The buckwheat is cooked once all the water has been absorbed.
8. Heat the olive oil in a frying pan when the tofu has 5 minutes left, heat the olive oil in a frying pan, when hot add the courgette, chili, celery, onion, ginger, and garlic and fry on high heat for two minutes, then reduce to medium heat for four minutes until the vegetables are cooked through but still crunchy. You will need to add a tablespoon of water if the vegetables start to stick to the pan. Add the tamari and kale and cook for another minute.
9. Serve with the greens and buckwheat when the tofu is ready.

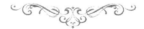

BUCKWHEAT NOODLES

Ingredients

- Shrimps, deveined and shelled, 1 ½ cup
- Extra virgin olive oil, 2 tsp
- Buckwheat noodles, 1 cup

- Soy sauce or tamari (gluten-free), 2 tsp
- 1 chopped garlic clove
- 1 chopped fresh ginger
- 1 freshly chopped bird's eye chili
- Chicken stock, 100 ml
- Sliced red onions, ½ cup
- Chopped kale, ½ cup
- Sliced and trimmed celery, ½ cup
- Celery leaves or lovage, 1 tsp
- Chopped green beans, 1 cup

Directions

Cook shrimps with 1 tsp of soy sauce or tamari and 1 tsp of olive oil for a couple of minutes on high heat. Pour the prawns out of the pan and wipe down oil residue with kitchen paper. Cook buckwheat noodles for up to eight minutes, drain and leave on the side to cool off. As your noodles cool down, fry the remaining ingredients (kale, beans, celery, ginger, red onion, chili, and garlic) up to three minutes. Add the stock to the mix and simmer for a couple more minutes. The vegetables should be cooked but still fresh-looking and crunchy. Finally, add the buckwheat noodles, celery, and prawns to the pan, boil briefly, and you're done.

MEAT

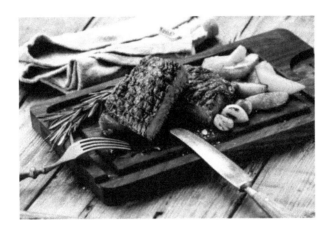

SIRTFOOD BEEF

Ingredients

- large beef steak
- diced potato
- Extra virgin olive oil, 1 tbsp
- Finely chopped parsley, ½ tbsp
- One sliced red onion
- Sliced kale, 1 cup
- Beef stock, 150 ml
- 1 finely chopped garlic clove
- Red wine, ½ cup
- Tomato sauce, 1 tsp
- 1 tbsp water
- Corn flour, 1 tsp

Directions

1. 1Preheat your oven to 220 ℃
2. Boil the potatoes in a saucepan for 4-5 minutes, transfer into the oven and roast for 30-45 with a little bit of olive oil. Turn every ten minutes so that the potatoes are roasted evenly. Pull out of the oven and add chopped parsley. Fry onions and garlic in a little bit of olive oil and add kale after a minute. Fry another two minutes until it turns soft.
3. Coat the meat in a thin layer of oil and fry on medium heat until it's cooked the way you like it. Remove from the pan add the wine into the remaining oil and leave to bubble. Once the wine is reduced by half and appears thicker, you can pour into the stock and tomato sauce and bring to a boil. Add corn flour paste until you achieve the desired consistency. Serve with the steak and vegetables.

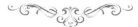

SIRTFOOD BEANS WITH BEEF

Ingredients

- Kidney beans, 2 small cans
- Lean beef, minced, 400 g
- Buckwheat, 160 g
- 1 finely chopped red onion
- 1 chopped red bell pepper
- Two finely chopped bird's eye chili peppers
- Canned tomatoes, 800 g
- Ground turmeric, 1 tbsp
- Tomato sauce, 1 tbsp
- Cocoa powder, 1 tbsp
- Ground cumin, 1 tbsp
- Extra virgin olive oil, 1 tbsp
- Red wine, 150 ml
- Chopped coriander, ½ tbsp.
- Chopped parsley, ½ tbsp.

Directions

4. Fry the onions, chili peppers, and garlic for three minutes over medium heat. Throw in the spices and mince for another minute. After that, add the beef and red wine. Bring to a boil and let it bubble until the liquid reduces by a half.
5. Add the cocoa powder, tomatoes, tomato sauce, and the red bell pepper. Add more water if needed and let the dish simmer on low medium heat for an hour. Add the remaining chopped herbs before serving.

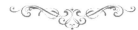

CHARGRILLED BEEF, A RED WINE JUS, ONION RINGS, GARLIC KALE, AND HERB ROASTED POTATOES

Planning time: 70 min. / Cooking time: 70 min. / Servings: 2

Ingredients

- 100g potatoes, stripped and dice
- 1 tablespoon extra-virgin olive oil
- 120–150g x 3.5cm-thick hamburger filet steak 40ml red wine 150ml meat stock
- 1 teaspoon tomato purée 1 teaspoon cornflour
- 1 tablespoon water
- 5g parsley, finely cleaved
- 50g red onion, cut into rings 50g kale, cut
- 1 garlic clove, finely cleaved ....

Directions

1. Preheat the oven to 220°C and place the potatoes in boiling water and cook for 4–5 minutes, channel. Pour 1 teaspoon oil in a simmering tin and meal the potatoes for 35–45 minutes turning the potatoes on each side like clockwork to guarantee they cook equitably.
2. Remove from the oven when completely cooked, sprinkle with cut parsley, and blend all together.
3. Pour 1 teaspoon of the oil on a pan and fry the onion for 5-7 minutes to turn out to be delicate and conveniently caramelized. Keep it warm.

4. Place the kale in a pan, steam for 2–3 minutes, and channel. In ½ teaspoon of oil, fry the garlic for 1 moment to turn out to be delicate however not hued. Add the kale and keep on singing for an additional 1–2 minutes to get delicate. Keep up the glow.

5. Over high warmth, place an ovenproof pan until it gets smoking. At that point utilize the ½ a teaspoon of the oil to cover the meat and fry over a medium-high warmth. Remove the meat and put aside to rest.

6. Pour the wine to the hot pan and air pocket to reduce the wine amount significantly to shape sweet and to have a concentrated flavor. Include the tomato purée and stock to the steak container and boil. Include the cornflour paste little at once to go about as a thickener to until the ideal consistency is accomplished. Include any juices from the refreshed steak and present with the kale, onion rings, cooked potatoes, and red wine sauce.

Nutrition: Calories: 244 kcal Protein: 14.26 g Fat: 14.46 g Sugars: 14.69 g

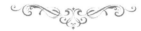

TURMERIC CHICKEN & KALE SALAD WITH HONEY LIME DRESSING-SIRTFOOD RECIPES

Planning time: 20 min. / Cooking time: 10 min. / Servings: 2

Ingredients

For the chicken

- 1 teaspoon ghee or 1 tbsp coconut oil
- ½ medium brown onion, diced
- 250-300 g / 9 oz. chicken mince or diced up chicken thighs
- 1 large garlic clove, finely diced
- 1 teaspoon turmeric powder
- 1 teaspoon lime zest
- juice of ½ lime
- ½ teaspoon salt + pepper

For the salad

- 6 broccolini stalks or 2 cups of broccoli florets

- 2 tablespoons pumpkin seeds (pepitas)
- 3 large kale leaves, stems removed and chopped
- ½ avocado, sliced
- handful of fresh coriander leaves, chopped
- handful of fresh parsley leaves, chopped

For the dressing

- 3 tablespoons lime juice
- 1 small garlic clove, finely diced or grated
- 3 tablespoons extra-virgin olive oil
- 1 teaspoon raw honey
- ½ teaspoon wholegrain or Dijon mustard
- ½ teaspoon sea salt and pepper

Directions

1. Heat the ghee or coconut oil in a small frying pan over medium-high heat. Add the onion and sauté on medium heat for 4-5 minutes, until golden. Add the chicken mince and garlic and stir for 2-3 minutes over medium-high heat, breaking it apart.
2. Add the turmeric, lime zest, lime juice, salt and pepper and cook, stirring frequently, for a further 3-4 minutes. Set the cooked mince aside.
3. While the chicken is cooking, bring a small saucepan of water to boil. Add the broccolini and cook for 2 minutes. Rinse under cold water and cut into 3-4 pieces each.
4. Add the pumpkin seeds to the frying pan from the chicken and toast over medium heat for 2 minutes, stirring frequently to prevent burning. Season with a little salt. Set aside. Raw pumpkin seeds are also fine to use.
5. Place chopped kale in a salad bowl and pour over the dressing. Using your hands, toss and massage the kale with the dressing. This will soften the kale, kind of like what citrus juice does to fish or beef carpaccio – it 'cooks' it slightly.
6. Finally toss through the cooked chicken, broccolini, fresh herbs, pumpkin seeds and avocado slices.

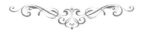

SIRTFOOD CHICKEN BREASTS

Prep Time: 0 hours 15 mins / Cook Time: 15 mins

Ingredients

- 120 g skinless, boneless chicken breast
- Two tsp. ground Tumeric juice of 1/4 lemon
- One tbsp. extra virgin olive oil
- 50 g kale, chopped
- Twenty g red onion, chopped
- One tsp. fresh ginger
- 50 g buckwheat
- For the Salsa:
- 130 g tomato
- One bird's eye chili, finely chopped
- One tbsp. capers, finely chopped
- Five g parsley, finely chopped juice of 1/4 lemon

Directions

To make the salsa, remove the eye from the tomato and chop it very finely, taking care to keep as much of the liquid as possible. Mix with the chili, capers, parsley, and lemon juice. You could put everything in a blender but the end result is a little different.

Heat the oven to 220°C/gas 7. Marinate the chicken breast in 1 teaspoon of turmeric, lemon juice, and a little oil. Leave for 5–10 minutes.

Heat an ovenproof frying pan until hot, then add the marinated chicken and cook for a minute or so on each side, until pale golden, then transfer to the oven (place on a baking tray if your pan isn't ovenproof) for 8–10 minutes or until cooked through. Remove from the oven, cover with foil, and leave to rest for 5 minutes before serving.

Meanwhile, cook the kale in a steamer for 5 minutes. Fry the red onions and the ginger in a little oil, until soft but not coloured, then add the cooked kale and fry for another minute.

Cook the buckwheat according to the packet instructions with the remaining teaspoon of turmeric. Serve alongside the chicken, vegetables, and salsa.

SWEET-SMELLING CHICKEN BREAST, KALE, RED ONION, AND SALSA

Planning time: 55 min / Cooking time: 30 min / Servings: 2

Ingredients

- 120g skinless, boneless chicken bosom 2 teaspoons ground turmeric
- 20g red onion, cut
- 1 teaspoon new ginger, sliced 50g buckwheat
- ¼ lemon
- 1 tablespoon extra-virgin olive oil 50 g kale, cleaved

Directions

1. To set up the salsa, remove the tomato eye and finely cut. Include the chili, parsley, capers, lemon juice, and blend.
2. Preheat the oven to 220°C. Pour 1 teaspoon of the turmeric, the lemon juice, and a little oil on the chicken bosom and marinate. Permit to remain for 5–10 minutes.
3. Place an ovenproof griddle on the warmth and cook the marinated chicken for a moment on each side to accomplish a pale brilliant color. At that point move the container containing the chicken to the oven and permit to remain for 8–10 minutes or until it is finished. Remove from the oven and spread with foil, put in a safe place for 5 minutes before serving.
4. Put the kale in a liner and cook for 5 minutes. Pour a little oil in a pan and fry the red onions and the ginger to turn out to be delicate yet not shaded. Include the cooked kale and keep on frying for another minute.
5. Cook the buckwheat adhering to the bundle's guidelines utilizing the rest of the turmeric. Serve close by the chicken, salsa, and vegetables.

Nutrition: Calories: 149 kcal, Protein: 15.85 g, Fat: 5.09 g, Sugars: 10.53 g

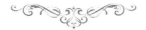

SINGED CHICKEN AND BROCCOLINI

Ingredients

- 2 tablespoons Coconut oil
- 400 g Chicken bosom Bacon blocks 150 g Broccolini 250 g

Directions

1. Cut the chicken into blocks.
2. Melt the coconut oil in a container over medium warmth and brown the chicken with the bacon solid shapes and cook through.
3. Season with chili drops, salt, and pepper. Include broccolini and fry.
4. Stack on a plate and appreciate!

Nutrition: Calories: 461 kcal Protein: 41.7 g Fat: 32.1 g Sugars: 4 g.

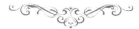

SAVORY CHICKEN WITH KALE AND RICOTTA SALAD

Ingredients

- Extra virgin olive oil, 1 tbsp
- 1 diced red onion
- 1 finely diced garlic cove
- Juice and zest from ½ lemon
- Diced chicken meat of your choosing, 300 g
- A pinch of salt
- A pinch of pepper

For salad

- Pumpkin seeds, 2 tbsp
- Finely chopped kale, 2 cup
- Ricotta cheese, ½ cup
- Coriander leaves, chopped, ¼ cup
- Parsley Leaves, chopped, ¼ cup

Salad dressing

- Orange juice, 3 tbsp

- 1 finely minced garlic clove
- Extra virgin olive oil, 3 tbsp
- Raw honey, 1 tsp
- Wholegrain mustard, ½ tsp
- A pinch of salt
- A pinch of pepper

Directions

1. Start by cooking chicken. Heat the oil over medium-high heat and add the onions. Let the onions sauté up to five minutes. Once the onions turn a golden color, add the chicken and garlic. If you'd like to finish quickly, stir-fry for up to three minutes at medium-high temperature, or lower the temperature and let it slowly simmer for up to fifteen minutes. The latter option will result in soft chicken, while the medium- heat stir fry will produce crunchy meat dices.
2. Next, add the lemon juice, pepper, zest, and turmeric during the last four minutes of cooking.
3. While your chicken is cooking, prepare the kale. While you can blanch the vegetable in boiling water up to two minutes, I'd recommend microwaving with ½ cup of water up to five minutes to preserve nutrients.
4. Remember, kale is edible raw, and cooking only serves to achieve the desired flavor and consistency. You can microwave the kale for as short as two minutes if all you need is for it to soften up, and the full five minutes if you prefer that fully-cooked taste.
5. During the last two minutes of chicken cooking, toss in the pumpkin seeds and stir fry. Remove from heat and set aside.

Mix both dishes into a bowl and add ricotta and the remaining fresh herbs. Enjoy

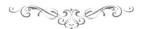

CHICKEN AND KALE BUCKWHEAT NOODLES

This tasty dish will take no more than 30 minutes to prepare, prep time included.

Ingredients

For noodles

- Finely chopped kale, 2 cup
- Buckwheat noodles, 5 oz
- Shiitake mushrooms (or any other of your choosing), four pieces
- Extra virgin olive oil, 1 tsp
- 1 finely diced red onion
- 1 diced chicken breast
- 1 sliced bird's eye chili
- Soy sauce, 3 tbsp

Salad dressing

- Soy sauce, ¼ cup
- Tamari sauce, 1 tbsp
- Sesame oil, 1 tbsp
- Lemon juice, 1 tbsp

Directions

1. Boil or stir-fry chicken for up to 15 minutes.
2. Microwave kale up to three minutes to preserve nutrients.
3. Cook buckwheat noodles and rinse and add kale once they're done.
4. Fry the mushrooms with 1 tsp of olive oil up to three minutes and season with a pinch of salt. Set aside and use the same pan, adding more olive oil, to sauté peppers and chickpeas up to five minutes. Add garlic, water, and tamari sauce, and cook for another three minutes. Add kale with noodles, chicken, and dressing. Mix all together and serve.

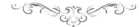

TURKEY WITH SIRTFOOD VEGETABLES

Ingredients

- Lean turkey meat, 150 g
- 1 finely chopped garlic clove
- 1 finely chopped red onion
- 1 finely chopped bird's eye chili/replace with chopped red bell paprika or ½ squeezed citrus fruit if you don't like spicy foods
- 1 tsp of finely chopped ginger

- Extra virgin olive oil, 2 tbsp
- Ground turmeric, 1 tbsp
- ½ cup of dried tomatoes
- Parsley, 10 g
- Sage, dried, 1 tsp
- ½ juiced lime or lemon
- Capers, 1 tbsp

Directions

1. Chop the cauliflower. Fry with chopped ginger, chili, red onion, and garlic in 1 tbsp olive oil until they're soft. Add cauliflower and turmeric, and cook for a couple of minutes until the cauliflower becomes soft. Once the dish is done, add dried tomatoes and parsley.
2. Coat your turkey in a thin layer of olive oil and sage. Fry for about five minutes, and then add the capers and lime juice to the mix. Add half a cup of water and bring to a boil

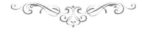

SIRTFOOD CAULIFLOWER COUSCOUS AND TURKEY STEAK

Planning time: 45 min / Cooking time: 10 min / Servings: 2

Ingredients

- 150 g cauliflower, generally cut 1 garlic clove, finely sliced
- 2 tsp ground turmeric
- 30 g sun-dried tomatoes, finely sliced 10g parsley
- 150 g turkey steak 1 tsp dried sage Juice of ½ lemon 1 tbsp tricks
- 40 g red onion, finely cut
- 1 bird's eye chili, finely sliced 1 tsp cleaved new ginger 2 tbsp additional virgin olive oil

Directions

1. Deteriorate the cauliflower utilizing a food processor. Mix in 1-2 heartbeats until the cauliflower has a breadcrumb-like consistency.
2. In a pan, fry garlic, stew, ginger, and red onion in 1 tsp olive oil for 2-3 minutes. Toss in the turmeric and cauliflower at that point cook for another 1-2 minutes. Remove from warmth and include the tomatoes and generally a large portion of the parsley.
3. Embellishment the turkey steak with wise and dress with oil. In a pan, over medium warmth, fry the turkey steak for 5 minutes, turning incidentally. When the steak is cooked include lemon juice, tricks, and a scramble of water. Mix and present with the couscous.

Nourishment: Calories: 462 kcal Protein: 16.81 g Fat: 39.86 g Starches: 9.94 g

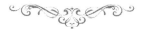

SIRTFOOD LAMB

Ingredients

- Extra virgin olive oil, 2 tbsp
- Grated ginger, one inch
- 1 sliced red onion.
- 1 tsp of bird's eye
- Cumin seeds, 2 tsp
- 1 cinnamon stick
- Lamb, 800 g
- Garlic cloves, crushed, 3 pieces
- A pinch of salt
- Chopped Medjool dates, 1 cup
- Chickpeas, 400 g
- Coriander, 2 tbsp
- Buckwheat

Directions

1. Start by preheating your oven to 140 °C. Sauté sliced onion with 2 tbsp of extra virgin olive oil for five minutes while keeping the lid on. The onions should turn soft but not brown.
2. Add turmeric, cumin, ginger, garlic, and chili and stir fry for another minute.
3. Add the chunks of lamb, season with salt and let, and let boil. Add a glass of water.
4. After the mixture has boiled, roast in the oven for one hour and 15 minutes. Add the chickpeas half an hour before the dish is finished.
5. Add chopped coriander and serve with buckwheat after the meal is done.

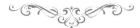

ROAST LAMB & RED WINE SAUCE

Planning time: 10 min / Cooking time: 10 min / Servings: 4

Ingredients

- 1.5kg (3lb 6oz) leg of lamb
- 5 cloves of garlic
- 6 sprigs of rosemary
- 3 tablespoons parsley
- 1 tablespoon honey
- 1 tablespoon olive oil
- ½ teaspoon sea salt
- 300mls (½ pint) red wine

Directions

Place the rosemary, garlic, parsley and salt into a pestle and mortar or small bowl and blend the ingredients together. Make small slits in the lamb and press a little of the mixture into each incision. Pour the oil over the meat and cover it with foil. Roast in the oven for around 1 hour 20 minutes.

Pour the wine into a small saucepan and stir in the honey. Warm the liquid then reduce the heat and simmer until reduced. Once the lamb is ready, pour the sauce over it, then return it to the oven to cook for another 5 minutes.

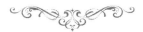

KALE AND RED ONION DHAL WITH BUCKWHEAT

Planning time 5 min / Cooking time 25 min / Servings: 2

Ingredients

- ½ tablespoon olive oil
- ½ little red onion, cut 1 ½ garlic cloves, squashed 1cm ginger, ground
- 100ml water
- 50g kale or spinach
- 80g buckwheat or brown rice
- ½ flying creatures eye chili, deseeded and finely cleaved 1 teaspoon turmeric
- 1 teaspoon garam masala 80g red lentils
- 200ml coconut milk ....

Directions

1. Warmth up the olive oil, include the cut onion, and cook on low warmth for 5 minutes until relaxed with the top on. At that point, include the ginger, garlic, and chili and keep cooking for an additional 1 moment.
2. Add to it, the garam masala, turmeric, and a sprinkle of water. Cook for 1 increasingly minute before including the coconut milk, red lentils, and 200ml water.
3. Altogether combine all and cook over a delicate warmth for 20 minutes with the top shut. At the point when the dhal begins staying, include somewhat more water and mix once in a while.
4. Include the kale, following 20 minutes and completely mix and still spread the cover to cook for an extra 5 minutes or 1-2 minutes when you substitute with spinach.
5. Put the buckwheat in a pan and pour boiling water like 15 minutes before the curry prepares. Permit the water to boil and cook for 10-12 minutes. Channel the buckwheat and present with the dhal.

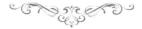

FISH

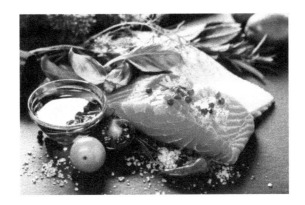

MATCHA GREEN TEA SALMON

Planning time: 10 min / Cooking time: 20 min / Servings: 3

Ingredients

- 4 (5 oz.) salmon fillets
- 2 tablespoons of extra virgin olive oil
- 2 tablespoons of fresh squeezed lemon juice
- 1 teaspoon of Matcha green tea powder
- ½ cup of wholegrain breadcrumbs
- Salt and pepper to taste

Directions

Preheat the oven to 350 degrees F.

While the oven is heating, add the olive oil, lemon juice, Matcha green tea powder, wholegrain breadcrumbs, salt and pepper to the large bowl and knead all the ingredients together using your hands.

Place the salmon fillets in the large bowl and cover them each with the breadcrumb mixture, pressing or patting into the fillet as needed. Place salmon fillets on a baking tray and bake them for 20 minutes.

SAVORY SIRTFOOD SALMON

Ingredients

- Salmon, 5 oz
- Lemon juice, 1 tbsp
- Ground turmeric, 1 tsp
- Extra virgin olive oil, 2 tbsp
- 1 chopped red onion
- 1 finely chopped garlic clove
- 1 finely chopped bird's eye chili
- Quinoa, 2 oz
- Finely chopped ginger, fresh, 1 tsp
- Celery, chopped, 1 cup
- Parsley, chopped, 1 tbsp
- Tomato, diced, 4.5 oz
- Vegetable stock, 100 ml

Directions

Preheat your oven to 200 ºC. Fry the celery, chili, garlic, onion, and ginger on olive oil up to three minutes. Add quinoa, tomatoes, and the chicken stock and let simmer for another ten minutes. Layer olive oil, lemon juice, and turmeric on top of the salmon and bake for ten minutes. Add parsley and celery before serving.

SALMON SIRT SUPER SALAD

Ingredients

- 50g chicory leaves
- 50g rocket
- 100g smoked salmon slices (you can also use tinned tuna or lentils, cooked chicken breast)
- 80g avocado, peeled, stoned and sliced
- 20g red onion, sliced
- 40g celery, sliced

- 15g walnuts, chopped
- 1 large Medjool date, pitted and chopped
- 1 tbs capers
- Juice ¼ lemon
- 1 tbs extra-virgin olive oil
- 10g lovage or celery leaves, chopped
- 10g parsley, chopped

Directions

Arrange the salad leaves on a plate. Mix all the ingredients together and serve on top of the leaves.

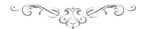

SIRTFOOD MISO SALMON

Ingredients

- Miso, ½ cup
- Organic red wine, 1 tbsp
- Extra virgin olive oil, 1 tbsp
- Salmon, 7 oz
- 1 sliced red onion
- Celery, sliced, 1 cup
- 2 finely chopped garlic cloves
- 1 finely chopped bird's eye chili
- Ground turmeric, 1 tsp
- Freshly chopped ginger, 1 tsp
- Green beans, 1 cup
- Kale, finely chopped, 1 cup
- Sesame seeds. 1 tsp
- Soy sauce, 1 tbsp
- Buckwheat, 2 tbsp

Directions

1. Marinate the salmon in the mix of red wine, 1 tsp of extra virgin olive oil, and miso for 30 minutes. Preheat your oven to 420 ⁰F and bake the fish for ten minutes.
2. Fry the onions, chili, garlic, green beans, ginger, kale, and celery for a few minutes until it's cooked. Insert the soy sauce, parsley, and sesame seeds.
3. Cook buckwheat per instructions and mix in with the stir-fry. Enjoy!

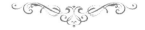

SIRTFOOD SALMON WITH KALE SALAD

Ingredients

- Salmon, 4 oz
- 2 sliced red onions
- Parsley, chopped, 1 oz
- Cucumber, 2 oz
- 2 sliced radishes
- Spinach, ½ cup
- Salad leaves, ½ cup

Salad dressing

- Raw honey, 1 tsp
- Greek yogurt, 1 tbsp
- Lemon juice, 1 tbsp
- Chopped mint leaves, 2 tbsp
- A pinch of salt
- A pinch of pepper

Directions

1. Preheat your oven to 200 ⁰C. Bake the salmon for up to 18 minutes and set aside. Mix in the ingredients for dressing and leave to sit between five and ten minutes.
2. Serve the salad with spinach and top with parsley, onions, cucumber, and radishes.

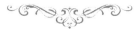

SHRIMP PASTA

Planning time 5 min / Cooking time 30 min / Servings: 3

Ingredients:

- 8 ounces linguine
- 1/4 cup mayonnaise
- 1/4 cup bean stew glue
- Two cloves garlic, squashes
- 1/2-pound shrimp, stripped
- One teaspoon salt
- 1/2 teaspoon cayenne pepper
- One teaspoon garlic powder
- One tablespoon vegetable oil
- One lime, squeezed
- 1/4 cup green onion, slashed
- 1/4 cup cilantro, minced
- Red bean stew chips, for embellish

Directions:

Cook pasta still somewhat firm as per box guidelines. In a little bowl, consolidate mayonnaise,
stew glue and garlic. Race to join. Put in a safe spot. In a blending bowl, include shrimp, salt,
cayenne and garlic powder. Mix to cover shrimp. Oil in a heavy skillet over medium warmth. Include shrimp and cook for around 2 minutes at that point flip and cook for an extra 2 minutes.
Add pasta and sauce to the dish. Mood killer the warmth and combine until the pasta is covered.
Include lime, green onions and cilantro, and topped with red bean stew pieces.

SIRTFOOD SHRIMPS WITH BUCKWHEAT NOODLES

Ingredients

- Shrimps (or a piece of fish of your choosing), 4 oz
- Tamari, 2 tbsp
- Extra virgin olive oil, 2 tbsp
- Buckwheat noodles, 75 g
- 1 finely chopped bird's eye chili
- 1 finely chopped garlic clove
- Fresh ginger, chopped, 1 tsp
- 1 sliced red onion
- Sliced red celery, ½ cup
- Chopped green beans, 1 cup
- Chopped kale, 1 cup
- Chicken stock, 1 cup
- Celery, 1 tsp

Directions

1. Cook the shrimps for three minutes on high heat and with 1 tsp of tamari and 1 tsp of extra virgin olive oil. Set aside.
2. Cook the noodles for up to eight minutes and set aside.
3. Fry kale, beans, celery, and onion, ginger, chili, and garlic in oil for up to three minutes. Add vegetable stock and simmer for two minutes.
4. Mix all together, bring to a boil, and serve.

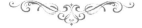

ASIAN SHRIMP STIR-FRY WITH BUCKWHEAT NOODLES

Ingredients

- ⅓ pound shelled raw jumbo shrimp, deveined
- Two teaspoons tamari (you can use soy sauce if you are not avoiding gluten)
- Two teaspoons extra virgin olive oil
- Three ounces (75g) soba (buckwheat noodles)
- Two garlic cloves, finely chopped
- One Thai chili, finely chopped
- One teaspoon finely chopped fresh ginger

- ½ cup (45g) celery including leaves, trimmed and sliced, with leaves set aside
- ½ cup (100ml) chicken stock
- ⅛ cup (20g) red onions, sliced
- ¾ cup (50g) kale, roughly chopped
- ½ cup (75g) green beans, chopped

Directions

1. Heat a frying pan over high heat. Cook the shrimp in one teaspoon of the tamari and 1 teaspoon of the oil for three minutes.
2. Transfer the shrimp to a plate. Wipe the pan out with a paper towel, as you are going to use it again.
3. Cook the noodles in boiling water for eight minutes or as directed on the package. Drain and set aside.
4. Meanwhile, fry the chili, ginger, garlic, red onion, celery (but not the leaves), green beans, and kale in the remaining tamari and oil over medium-high heat for two to Three minutes. Add the stock and take to a boil, then simmer for a minute or two, until the vegetables are cooked but still crunchy.
5. Add the noodles, celery leaves, and shrimp to the pan, bring back to a boil, then remove from the heat and serve.

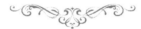

SIRTFOOD SHRIMP NOODLES

Ingredients

- Shrimps, deveined ⅓ lb
- Soy sauce, 2 tsp
- Extra virgin olive oil, 2 tsp
- Buckwheat noodles, 3oz
- 2 finely chopped garlic cloves
- 1 bird's eye chili, finely chopped
- Chopped fresh ginger, 1 tsp
- Chopped red onion, ¼
- Chopped celery with eaves, ½ cup
- Chopped green beans, ½ cup
- Chopped kale, 1 cup
- Chicken stock, ½ cup

Directions

- Cook the shrimps in 1 tsp of the soy sauce and one tsp of the oil up to three minutes on high heat.
- Cook buckwheat noodles for up to eight minutes and drain.
- Fry the remaining ingredients in a pan on medium heat for up to three minutes. Add the chicken stock, bring to a boil, and cook until the veggies are cooked, but still look fresh. Add the shrimps and noodles, bring to a boil, and you're done.

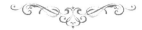

FISH SALAD

Planning time: 30 min / Cooking time: 0 min / Servings: 2

Ingredients

- 100g red chicory
- 2 hard-boiled eggs, stripped and quartered 2 tomatoes, cleaved
- 2 tbsp new parsley, cleaved 1 red onion, cut
- 150g fish pieces in brackish water, depleted 100g cucumber
- 1 celery stem
- 1 tbsp tricks
- 2tbsp garlic vinaigrette
- 25g rocket
- 6 kalamata olives, pitted

Directions

Consolidate all ingredients in a bowl and serve.

1. Top the fish with the infused oil, dill, and scallion and serve with the mango sauce, nuts, lime, and cilantro.

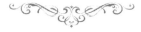

SIRTFOOD SHELLFISH SALAD

Ingredients

- Tomato sauce, 1 tsp
- Cloves, ¼ tsp
- Coriander, chopped, 1 tbsp
- Parsley, chopped, 1 tbsp
- Lemon juice, 1 tbsp (½ of a lemon)
- Kale, chopped, 1 cup
- Spinach, chopped, 1 cup
- Sea fruit of your choosing (shrimps, prawns, or clamps), 1 cup
- Chopped firm tofu, 1 thick slice (approx. 4 oz)
- Buckwheat noodles, 1 cup
- Pecan nuts, ½ cup
- Chopped ginger, ½ cup
- Miso paste, 1 tbsp
- Carrots, ½ cup
- Chicken stock, 100 ml

Directions

Simmer tomato sauce with lemon juice, chicken stock, coriander, parsley, and shrimps/cloves/clams for 10 minutes on medium heat. Add the remaining ingredients without the ginger and miso, and stir-fry until the shellfish is cooked through. Add the remaining seasonings, and you're done!

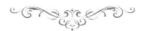

FISH WITH MANGO AND TURMERIC

Ingredients

- A fresh 1 ¼ lbs piece of fish of your choosing
- ½ cup of coconut oil
- A pinch of sea salt
- 1 tbsp of high-quality red wine
- ¼ cup olive oil
- ½ tbsp minced ginger

- Scallion, 2 cup
- Dill, 2 cup
- 1 ripe mango
- 1 squeezed lemon
- 1 garlic clove
- Dry red pepper, 1 tsp
- Fresh cilantro
- Walnuts

Directions

2. Marinate the fish and leave overnight
3. Blend the ingredients for mango dipping sauce
4. Fry the fish in 2 tbsp in coconut oil on medium heat and add a pinch of salt after five minutes. Turn to the other side and fry for another couple of minutes. Keep the remaining oil in the pan. Add scallions and dill and turn off the heat. Heat for about 15 seconds and season with a pinch of salt.

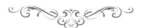

SNACKS

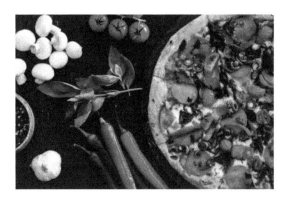

SIRTFOOD PIZZA 1

Sirtfood Pizzas are delicious and satiating, aside from being low-carb, low-calorie, and nutrient- rich. While you don't have to bake entirely Sirtfood pizzas to follow this diet plan, and instead you can just add individual Sirtfoods to your favorite pizza, these recipes will fit into your 1,000-1,500 daily calorie limit. Here's how to bake two small Sirtfood pizzas:

Ingredients

Base

- Flour, 14 oz (½ buckwheat flour, ½ rice or white flour)
- Water, 3 cup
- 1 bag of dried yeast
- 1 tbsp of extra virgin olive oil
- 1 tsp of brown sugar

Sauce

- 14 oz of chopped tomatoes, fresh or canned
- ½ chopped red onion
- 1 chopped garlic clove
- 2 tbsp of red wine

- 1 tsp of extra virgin olive oil
- Dried oregano, 1 tsp
- Basil leaves, 1 tsp

Toppings

- Grilled eggplant, red onion, arugula
- Cherry tomato, chili flakes, cottage cheese or mozzarella
- Olives, cooked chicken
- Kale (fresh and steamed), chorizo, mushrooms, red onion

Directions

1. Start off by making the dough. First, dissolve the yeast in water and add sugar. Leave up to 15 minutes covered in clingfilm.
2. Next, slowly pour the flour into the bowl. Pay attention not to create clumps as you pour the flour into the yeast.
3. Add the extra virgin olive oil and start mixing the dough. Proceed to knead until the mix is smooth, consistent, and thick.
4. Leave the dough to rise up to 60 minutes in an oiled bowl, after you've covered it with a damp cloth or a tea towel. You'll know the dough has risen enough when it doubles in size.
5. While your dough rises, start making your sauce. Start by frying chopped garlic and onion in a small dose of olive oil. Once the onion softens, pour in the wine and add dried oregano. Proceed cooking until the mixture reduces by half.
6. Add chopped tomatoes, stir, and pour the sugar into the sauce. Proceed cooking for another 30 minutes. Wait until your dough rises and knead for a couple more minutes to remove the air bubbles. Heat your oven to 220 °C. Dust your kitchen counter with flour, split the dough into halves, and roll out the pieces until you like their thickness. Transfer onto the baking tray or the pizza stone.
7. Now layer the tomato sauce over the dough and leave a small gap along the edges. Add the toppings you like, and in quantities you prefer. However, make sure to add any heat sensitive ingredients, like arugula or chili, after you've baked the pizza. Leave for another 15 minutes for the dough to start rising again. Bake for up to 12 minutes. Once your pizza is out of the oven, add fresh herbs and toppings of your choosing.

Great job! You now know which meals to cook during your Sirtfood diet calorie restriction. Rest assured that these recipes will help you feel full and energized throughout the entire day. Here are some general tips and tricks for more convenient

Sirtfood cooking:

- **Be practical.** Most of the recipes given in this chapter won't take longer than 30-45 minutes to make. However, you can make the process even faster and easier by pre- making meals the day or night before, or cooking larger amounts of meat and vegetables and storing your meals in the fridge.

- **Invest in quality pots.** Quality cooking supplies guarantee that you'll be able to stir-fry without using a lot of oil. The majority of recipes given in this chapter are easy to cook with no more than 2 tbsp of extra virgin olive oil. But, without the right dishes, it could happen that your foods start to stick to the bottom of the pan. In this case, instead of adding more oil, simply pour a little bit of water.

- **Substitutes**. Don't like some of the ingredients provided in these recipes? Or, you find some of them difficult to find or expensive to purchase? Don't worry! Each of these meals can be adjusted according to your taste. Here are a couple of substitutes that you can use for some of the ingredients:

  - **Meat**. You can substitute different types of meat for an equal amount of any other meat you like. You can also substitute meat with mushrooms, potatoes, eggs, and beans.

  - **Fruit**. If you don't want to use avocados, you can replace them with bananas or melons. Melons have a similar consistency, and while they don't taste the same as avocados, they won't significantly alter a dish.

  - **Buckwheat**. As you may have noticed, buckwheat is heavily featured in the majority of recipes. If you don't want to eat that much of it, you can switch it with an equal amount of quinoa, kale, spinach, or beans. Keep in mind that doing so will affect the steps in cooking, and may affect preparation time. If you're not using leafy greens to substitute buckwheat, but you're using beans or legumes instead, it would be the best to cook the substitutes beforehand, and add them to other dishes as they're being cooke.

SIRTFOOD PIZZA 2

Makes 2 x 30cm pizzas

For the pizza base

- 1 x 7g packet of dried yeast
- 300ml lukewarm water
- One tsp brown sugar

- 200g strong pasta flour or white flour plus a little extra for rolling out
- 200g buckwheat flour
- One tbsp extra virgin olive oil, plus a little extra for greasing

For the tomato sauce

- ½ red onion, finely chopped
- One garlic clove, finely chopped
- One tsp extra virgin olive oil
- One tsp dried oregano
- Pinch of brown sugar
- Two tbsp white wine
- 5g basil leaves
- 1 x 400g tin of chopped tomatoes

Some favorite toppings for your Sirtfood Pizza

- Red onion, grilled aubergine, and Rocket – buy it from a deli, or griddle 3-5mm slices of aubergine brushed with extra virgin olive oil until it has black grill marks on either side and is soft.
- Cherry tomato, goat's cheese, chilli flakes, and rocket
- Cooked chorizo, red onion and steamed kale
- Cooked chicken, rocket, red onion and olives

Directions

1. For the dough, dissolve the sugar and yeast in the water. Cover with clingfilm and leave for ten to fifteen minutes.
2. Sift the flour in a bowl. Fit it with the dough hook if you have a stand mixer, and sift the flour into the mixer bowl. Add the yeast mixture and oil to the flour and blend together to form a dough.
3. Knead until smooth and springy, then move to an oiled cup, cover with a clean damp tea towel and allow to rise for fifty minutes somewhere warm, until doubled in size.
4. In the meantime, make your tomato sauce. Fry the garlic and onion in the olive oil until soft, add the dried oregano and bubble and wine to reduce it by half.
5. Add the sugar and tomatoes, then bring to a boil, and cook until thick. Remove from the heat. To extract the air, knead the dough over again. Heat up the furnace to 230C/gas 8. Dust a work surface gently with flour. Cut the dough in half and roll out each piece to the thickness you need and put it on a pizza stone or non-stick oiled baking tray.

6. Spread a thin layer of tomato sauce over the dough (you'll only need about half the sauce for this quantity of dough but can freeze any left-over), leaving a space around the edge for the crust. If you're using rocket and chili flakes, add the rest of your ingredients after you've baked your pizza.
7. Set aside for twenty minutes before baking, the dough will start to rise again, giving a lighter base.
8. Bake for twelve minutes.

Enjoy your Sirtfood Pizza!

Chapter 8
VEGETARIAN SIRT FOOD RECIPES

BREAKFAST

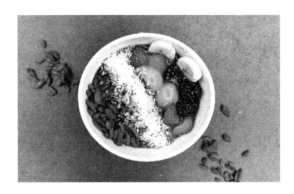

STRAWBERRY BUCKWHEAT PANCAKES

Planning time: 5 Min / Cooking Time: 45 Min / Servings 4

Ingredients

- 3½oz strawberries, cleaved 3½ oz buckwheat flour
- 1 teaspoon olive oil
- 1 teaspoon olive oil for fricasseeing Freshly crushed juice of 1 orange
- 1 egg
- 8fl oz milk

Directions

1. Empty the milk into a bowl and blend in the egg and a teaspoon of olive oil. Filter in the flour to the fluid blend until smooth and velvety. Permit it to rest for 15 minutes. Warmth a little oil in a dish and pour in a fourth of the blend or to the size you like.

2. Sprinkle in a fourth of the strawberries into the hitter. Cook for around 2 minutes on each side. Serve hot with a sprinkle of juice orange. You could have a go at exploring different avenues regarding different berries, for example, blueberries and blackberries.
Nourishment: Calories: 180 kcal, Protein: 7.46 g, Fat: 7.5 g Starches: 22.58 g.

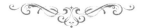

BUCKWHEAT APPLE PANCAKES

This recipe will give your four quick, healthy, and delicious pancakes.

Ingredients

- Two eggs
- Buckwheat flour, 2 cup
- Sugar, 2 tbsp
- A pinch of salt
- Two chopped, peeled apples
- Skim milk, 3 cup
- Olive oil, 2 tsp
- Baking powder, 1 tsp

Directions

1. Cook apples in a small amount of water, up to ½ cup and let boil up to two minutes. Blend to create a sauce.
2. Now, start making pancakes. Mix baking powder, the flour, and sugar into a bowl.
3. Add milk and mix until the texture is even and smooth. Mix in both eggs.
4. Fry ¼ of the batter on ½ tsp of olive oil on medium high heat. Repeat four times, until you fry all of the batter.

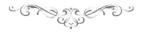

FLAPJACKS WITH APPLES AND BLACKCURRANTS

Planning time: 5 Min / Cooking Time: 50 Min / Servings 4

Ingredients

- 2 apples, cut into little pieces 2 cups of fast cooking oats
- 1 cup flour of your decision 1 tsp preparing powder
- 2 egg whites
- 1 ¼ cups of milk or soy/rice/coconut 2 tsp additional virgin olive oil
- A scramble of salt
- 2 tbsp. crude sugar, coconut sugar, or 2 tbsp. nectar that is warm and simple to appropriate

For the berry beating:

- 1 cup blackcurrants, washed and follows evacuated 3 tbsp. water may utilize less
- 2 tbsp. sugar see above for types

Directions

1. Place the elements for the garnish in a little pot stew, mixing now and again for around 10 minutes until it cooks down and the juices are discharged.
2. Take the dry ingredients and blend in a bowl. After, include the apples and the milk a piece at a time you may not utilize everything), until it is a hitter. Firmly whisk the egg whites and afterward tenderly blend them into the hotcake player. Put aside in the cooler.
3. Pour a one-fourth of the oil onto a level dish or level frying pan, and when hot, empty a portion of the player into it in a flapjack shape. At the point when the flapjacks begin to have brilliant brown edges and structure air boils, they might be prepared to be tenderly flipped.
4. Test to be certain the base can live away from the dish before really flipping. Repeat for the following three hotcakes. Top every flapjack with the berries.

Nutrition: Calories: 470 kcal, Protein: 11.71 g, Fat: 16.83 g Sugars: 79 g.

SIRTFOOD FRUIT YOGURT

Ingredients

- Strawberries, chopped, 1 cup
- Raspberries, 1 cup
- Greek yogurt, 2 cup
- Chia seeds, 1 tbsp

Directions

Blend the berries with Greek yogurt and chia seeds and enjoy!

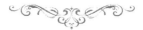

VEGETARIAN SIRTFOOD OMELET

Ingredients

- 2 eggs
- Kale, chopped, ½ cup
- Ground turmeric, 1 tsp
- Ginger, finely chopped, 1 tsp
- 1 sliced bird's eye chili
- Extra virgin olive oil, 1 tsp

Directions

Mix all ingredients together. Optionally, you can blend for a minute if you prefer a homogenous- looking omelet. Fry in olive oil. First, layer the eggs across the frying pan and wait for the edges to turn dry and golden. Flip and fry on the other side.

EGGS AND SIRTFOOD VEGETABLES

Ingredients

- 1 egg
- Kale, chopped, 1 cup
- Chopped parsley, 1 tbsp
- Chopped red onion, ½ cup
- Extra virgin olive oil, 1 tsp
- 1 finely chopped garlic clove
- Finely chopped celery, ½ cup
- 1 finely chopped paprika or bird's eye chili
- Ground turmeric, 1 tsp
- Ground cumin, 1 tsp
- Paprika, 1 tsp
- 1 14 oz can of sliced tomatoes

Directions

Fry the chili, spices, garlic, onion, and celery for a minute or two in olive oil, add the tomato sauce and let it simmer for 20 minutes. Pop the kale into the pan and cook for another five minutes, adding more water as needed. Lastly, add the parsley. Break the eggs and stir into the sauce, or boil them and serve next to the sauce.

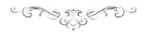

LUNCH

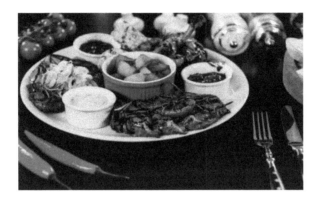

SINGED CAULIFLOWER RICE

Planning time: 55 min. / Cooking time: 10 min. / Servings 2

Ingredients

- piece Cauliflower
- tablespoon Coconut oil 1 piece Red onion
- 4 cloves Garlic
- ½ pieces Carrot
- ½ pieces Red chime pepper
- ½ pieces Lemon (the juice)
- 2 tablespoon pumpkin seeds
- 2 tablespoon new coriander
- 60 ml Vegetable stock
- 1.5 cm new ginger
- 1 teaspoon Chili drops

Directions

1. Cut the cauliflower into little rice grains in a food processor.
2. Finely slice the onion, garlic and ginger, cut the carrot into meager strips, dice the ringer pepper and finely cleave the herbs.

3. Dissolve 1 tablespoon of coconut oil in a pan and include half of the onion and garlic to the container and fry quickly until translucent.
4. Include cauliflower rice and season with salt.
5. Pour in the stock and mix everything until it dissipates and the cauliflower rice is delicate.
6. Remove the rice from the dish and put it in a safe place.
7. Dissolve the remainder of the coconut oil in the pan and include the rest of the onions, garlic, ginger, carrots, and peppers.
8. Fry for a couple of moments until the vegetables are delicate. Season them with somewhat salt.
9. Include the cauliflower rice once more, heat the entire dish, and include the lemon juice. Enhancement with pumpkin seeds and coriander before serving.

Nourishment: Calories: 230 kcal, Protein: 5.13 g, Fat: 17.81 g Starches: 17.25 g.

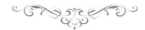

SIRTFOOD LENTILS

Planning time: 55 min. / Cooking time: 50 min. / Servings 2

Ingredients

- 1 cup chopped cherry tomatoes
- Extra virgin olive oil, 2 tsp
- 1 finely chopped red onion
- 1 finely chopped garlic clove
- Celery, thin-sliced, ½ cup
- Carrots, diced, ½ cup
- Paprika or bird's eye chili, 1 tsp
- Thyme, dry or fresh, 1 tsp
- Parsley, 1 tbsp
- Arugula, 20 g
- Chopped kale, 1 cup
- Lentils, 1 cup
- Vegetable stock, 220 ml

Directions

1. Preheat your oven to 120 °C
2. Roast the tomatoes for 30 minutes
3. Stir-fry paprika/bird-eye chili, garlic, red onion, carrot, and celery on 1 tsp olive oil. Once the vegetables have softened, add paprika and thyme. Add vegetable stock. Cook for another minute or two. Rinse your lentils and add to the pan until the mixture boils. Reduce the heat and simmer lightly for another 20 minutes. Stir regularly and add water if you feel like the mix is becoming too dry.
4. Add kale to the mix, wait another 10 minutes, and stir in roasted tomatoes and parsley. Top with fresh arugula and drizzle with lemon juice and olive.

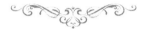

HOT CHICORY & NUT SALAD

Planning time: 5 min / Cooking time:40 min / Servings 2

Ingredients

For the salad:

- 100g 3½ oz green beans
- 100g 3½ oz red chicory, chopped if unavailable use yellow chicory
- 100g 3½ oz celery, chopped
- 25g 1oz macadamia nuts, chopped
- 25g 1oz walnuts, chopped
- 25g 1oz plain peanuts, chopped
- 2 tomatoes, chopped
- 1 tablespoon olive oil

For the dressing:

- 2 tablespoons fresh parsley, finely chopped
- ½ teaspoon turmeric
- ½ teaspoon mustard
- 1 tablespoon olive oil

- 25mls 1fl oz red wine vinegar
- 438 calories per serving

Directions

1. Mix together the ingredients for the dressing then set them aside. Heat a tablespoon of olive oil in a frying pan then add the green beans, chicory and celery.
2. Cook until the vegetables have softened then add in the chopped tomatoes and cook for 2 minutes. Add the prepared dressing, and thoroughly coat all of the vegetables.
3. Serve onto plates and sprinkle the mixture of nuts over the top. Eat immediately.

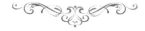

EGGS WITH ZUCCHINI AND ONIONS

Ingredients

- 4 eggs
- Olive oil, 1 tsp
- 1 finely chopped onion
- 1 red chili pepper, finely chopped
- 1 finely chopped garlic clove
- 1 finely chopped zucchini
- Tomato sauce, 1 tbsp
- A pinch of salt
- A pinch of Bird's eye chili powder
- A pinch of ground cumin
- Chopped tomatoes, 14 oz
- Canned quinoa, 14 oz
- Chopped parsley, ⅓ oz

Directions

4. Fry onions and peppers up to five minutes in a thin layer of oil in a saucepan on low temperature. Add the zucchini and garlic, bring to a boil, and then add tomato sauce, salt, and spices. Stir and add quinoa and chopped tomatoes. Increase the heat to medium-high and let simmer for 30 minutes until the sauce reduces by a third.

5. Remove from the stove, add chopped parsley, and preheat your oven to 200 °C. Add the eggs to the dish without stirring, cover with foil, and bake up to 15 minutes.

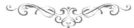

TOMATO FRITTATA

Planning time: 55 min / Cooking time:20 min / Servings 2

Ingredients:

- 50 g cheese, ground
- tbsp new parsley, cleaved 1 tbsp new basil, cut
- 1 tbsp olive oil
- 75 g kalamata olives, pitted and divided 8 cherry tomatoes, split
- 4 enormous eggs

Directions

1. Whisk eggs together in an enormous blending bowl. Hurl in the parsley, basil, olives, tomatoes, and cheese, blending all.
2. In a little pan, heat the olive oil over high warmth. Pour in the frittata blend and cook for 5-10 minutes, or set. Remove the pan from the hob and place under the flame broil for 5 minutes, or until firm and set. Partition into segments and serve right away.

Nourishment: Calories: 269 kcal, Protein: 9.23 g, Fat: 23.76 g Starches: 5.49 g.

TOMATO AND BUCKWHEAT SALAD

Ingredients

- Buckwheat noodles, 12 cup
- Arugula, 1 cup
- Basil leaves, 2 pieces
- 1 large chopped tomato
- Grilled tofu, 1 slice, chopped
- Olives, 12 cups

- Walnuts, ½ cup
- Extra virgin olive oil, 1 tbsp
- Lemon juice, 1 tbsp

Directions

Cook buckwheat noodles per instructions on the packaging. Mix the remaining ingredients together to make a salad. Add drained buckwheat noodles and drizzle with the olive oil and the lemon juice.

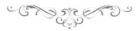

GRILLED MUSHROOM AND TOFU SUMMER SALAD

Ingredients

- Black olives, ½ cup
- 1 chopped tomato
- 1 chopped Bird's eye chili pepper
- Sliced red onion, ½
- 1 sliced cucumber
- Grilled tofu, cubed, 1 cup
- Mushrooms of your choosing, 2 cup
- Parsley, 1 tsp
- Basil, 1 tsp
- Ginger (optional), 1 tsp

Directions

1. Grill mushrooms and tofu on a thin layer of olive oil for up to five minutes. Mushrooms can, but don't have to be fully fried, depending on the type.
2. Next, mix in the remaining vegetables and add the freshly fried mushrooms with tofu. Mix all together, add parsley, basil, and ginger, and drizzle with lemon juice and olive oil.

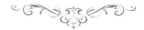

SIRTFOOD TOFU SESAME SALAD

Ingredients

- Sesame seeds, 1 tbsp
- 1 sliced cucumber
- Kale, chopped, 1 cup
- Arugula, 1 cup
- 1 fine sliced red onion
- Chopped parsley, ¼ cup
- Grilled tofu, diced, 2 cups
- Extra virgin olive oil, 2 tbsp
- Lime juice, 2 tbsp
- Soy sauce, 2 tbsp
- Raw honey, 1 tsp

Directions

1. First, start by roasting sesame seeds for up to two minutes. Set aside to cool. If you've bought raw tofu, grill briefly on a thin layer of olive oil. Leave the remaining oil for salad dressing.
2. Mix vegetables and spices into a bowl. Toss in the chopped grilled tofu and sesame seeds, and mix to distribute evenly throughout the salad. To finish off, drizzle with lime juice and olive oil.

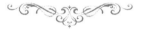

SWEET ARUGULA AND SALMON SALAD

Ingredients

- Arugula, ½ cup
- Chicory leaves, ½ cup
- Lentils, 1 cup
- 1 sliced red onion
- Sliced avocado, 80 g
- Sliced celery, ½ cup
- Chopped walnuts, 1 tbsp

- 1 pitted, chopped, Medjool date
- Extra virgin olive oil, 1 tbsp
- Lime juice, 1 tbsp
- Chopped parsley, 1 tbsp
- Celery leaves, chopped, 1 tbsp

Directions

Mix all ingredients into a bowl. Drizzle with lime juice and olive oil, spread on a large plate, and enjoy!

DINNER

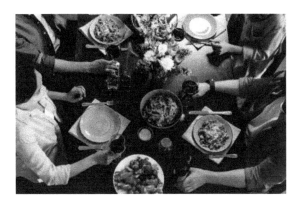

FRITTATA WITH SPRING ONIONS AND ASPARAGUS

Planning time: / Cooking time: / Servings: 2

Ingredients

- 5 pieces Egg
- 100 g Asparagus tips 4 pieces Spring onions 1 teaspoon Tarragon
- 1 juice Chili drops
- 80 ml Almond milk
- 2 tablespoon Coconut oil 1 clove Garlic

Directions

1. Preheat the oven to 220 ° C.
2. Crush the garlic and finely slice the spring onions.
3. Whisk the eggs with the almond milk and season with salt and pepper.
4. Melt 1 tablespoon of coconut oil in a medium-sized cast iron dish and quickly fry the onion and garlic with the asparagus.

5. Remove the vegetables from the container and liquefy the rest of the coconut oil in the dish.
6. Pour in the egg blend and half of the whole vegetable.
7. Place the pan in the oven for 15 minutes until the egg has cemented.
8. At that point remove the pan from the oven and pour the remainder of the egg with the vegetables into the container.
9. Place the pan in the oven again for 15 minutes until the egg is overall quite free. Sprinkle the tarragon and chili drops on the dish before serving.

Nourishment: Calories: 464 kcal, Protein: 24.23 g, Fat: 37.84 g Starches: 7.33 g.

BUCKWHEAT NOODLES WITH TOMATO AND SHRIMP

Ingredients

- Raw shrimps, 2 cup
- Buckwheat noodles, 1 cup
- Extra virgin olive oil, 1 tbsp
- One finely chopped garlic clove
- One finely chopped red onion
- Finely chopped celery, ¼ of a cup
- One finally chopped bird's eye chili
- Organic red wine, 2 tbsp
- Tomato sauce, 4 cup
- Chopped parsley, 1 tbsp

Directions

Fry the garlic, onions, chili and celery in extra virgin olive oil for two minutes over medium heat. Add the red wine and tomato sauce and cook for another 30 minutes. Add water if needed. Prepare the buckwheat noodles while the sauce is cooking. Add pasta to the sauce when cooked. And the shrimps and cook for another four minutes. When the dish is cooked, add chopped parsley and serve.

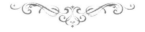

ROAST BALSAMIC VEGETABLES

Planning time: 35 Min. /Cooking time: 50 Min. /Servings: 2

Ingredients

- 4 tomatoes, chopped
- 2 red onions, chopped
- 3 sweet potatoes, peeled and chopped 100g (3½ oz) red chicory (or if unavailable, use yellow)
- 100g (3½ oz) kale, finely chopped 300 g (11 oz) potatoes, peeled and chopped 5 stalks of celery,
- chopped
- 1 bird s-eye chilli, de-seeded and finely chopped 2 tablespoons fresh parsley, chopped 2
- tablespoons fresh coriander (cilantro) chopped 3 tablespoons olive oil
- 2 tablespoons balsamic vinegar 1 teaspoon mustard
- Sea salt
- Freshly ground black pepper

Directions

Place the olive oil, balsamic, mustard, parsley and coriander (cilantro) into a bowl and mix well.

Toss all the remaining ingredients into the dressing and season with salt and pepper. Transfer the

vegetables to an ovenproof dish and cook in the oven at 200C/400F for 45 minutes.

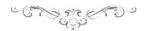

MEXICAN BELL PEPPER FILLED WITH EGG

Planning time: 55 min / Cooking time: 20 min / Servings 2

Ingredients

- 1 tablespoon Coconut oil 4 pieces Egg
- 1 piece Tomato
- 1 piece green peppers
- 2 tablespoon new coriander
- 1 juice Chili drops
- ¼ teaspoon ground cumin ¼ teaspoon Paprika powder ½ pieces Avocado

Directions

1. Cut the tomatoes and avocado into shapes and finely cut the new coriander.
2. Melt the coconut oil in a pan over medium warmth, beat the eggs in the container, and include the tomato solid shapes.
3. Continue blending until the egg cement and season with chili, caraway, paprika, pepper, and salt.
4. At long last include the avocado.
5. Place the egg blend in the pepper parts and enhancement with new coriander.

Nourishment: Calories: 497 kcal, Protein: 20.91 g, Fat: 41.27 g Starches: 14.41 g.

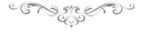

ONION MUSHROOM SALSA

Ingredients

- Mushrooms, 1 ⅓ cups
- Ground turmeric, 2 tsp
- Lime juice, 1 tbsp

- Chopped Kale, 1 cup
- 1 sliced red onion
- Arugula, 1 cup
- Fresh ginger, chopped, 1 ts

Directions

Fry the mushrooms on a thin layer of extra virgin olive oil for up to five minutes, while stirring and making sure they're cooking evenly. As you fry, sprinkle turmeric over the mushrooms. Add kale half-way through, letting it soften only lightly. Prepare a plate and lay out fresh arugula.

Mix the remaining ingredients together to make a salsa. If you'd like a more sauce-like consistency, you can blend the vegetables, spices, and the remaining oil. Serve one dish next to another and enjoy!

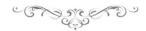

DISH WITH SPINACH AND EGGPLANT

Planning time: 1 hour / Cooking time: 40 min / Servings: 2

Ingredients

- Olive oil 3 tablespoon Spinach (new) 450 g Tomatoes 4 pieces
- Egg 2 pieces
- 1 piece Eggplant
- 2 teaspoons Lemon juice
- 4 tablespoon Almond flour
- 2 pieces Onion
- 60 ml Almond milk

Directions

1. Preheat the oven to 200 ° C.
2. Cut the eggplants, onions, and tomatoes into cuts and sprinkle salt on the eggplant cuts.
3. Brush the eggplants and onions with olive oil and fry them in a barbecue pan. Shrink the spinach in an enormous pan over moderate warmth and channel in a sifter.
4. Put the vegetables in layers in a lubed heating dish: first the eggplants, at that point the spinach and afterward the onion and the tomato. Repeat this.

5. Whisk eggs with almond milk, lemon juice, salt, and pepper and pour over the vegetables.
6. Sprinkle almond flour over the dish and heat in the oven for around 30 to 40 minute.
Nutrition: Calories: 446 kcal, Protein: 13.95 g, Fat: 31.82 g Sugars: 30.5 g.

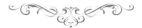

VEGGIE LOVER PALEO RATATOUILLE

Planning time: 70 min. / Cooking time: 55 min. / Servings 2

Ingredients

- 200 g Tomato solid shapes (can) 1/2 pieces Onion
- 2 cloves Garlic
- 1 piece hot peppers
- 1 teaspoon dried thyme
- 1/4 teaspoon dried oregano
- 1/4 TL Chili drops 2 tablespoon Olive oil 1 piece Eggplant
- 1 piece Zucchini

Directions

1. Preheat the oven to 180 ° C and gently oil a round or oval shape. Finely slice the onion and garlic.
2. Blend the tomato shapes with garlic, onion, oregano and stew chips, season with salt and pepper, and put on the base of the preparing dish.
3. Utilize a mandolin, a cheese slicer or a sharp blade to cut the eggplant, zucchini and hot pepper into dainty cuts.
4. Put the vegetables in a bowl (make hovers, start at the edge and work inside).
5. Shower the staying olive oil on the vegetables and sprinkle with thyme, salt, and pepper.
6. Spread the preparing dish with a bit of material paper and heat in the oven for 45 to 55 minutes.
Nourishment: Calories: 273 kcal, Protein: 5.66 g, Fat: 14.49 g Starches: 35.81 g.

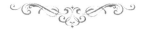

VEGAN CURRY FROM THE CROCK-POT

Planning time: 6 hours / Cooking time: 6 hours / Servings: 2

Ingredients

- 100 ml Vegetable stock 400 g Tomato shapes (can) 250 g Sweet peas
- 2 tablespoon tapioca flour
- 2 tablespoon Curry powder
- 1 teaspoon Ground caraway (ground) ¼ teaspoon Chili powder
- 4 pieces Carrot
- 2 pieces Sweet potato 1 piece Onion
- 3 cloves Garlic
- 1/4 TL Celtic ocean salt
- 1 juice Cinnamon

Directions

1. Generally cut vegetables and potatoes and press garlic. Divide the sugar snap peas.
2. Put the carrots, yams, and onions in the moderate cooker.
3. Blend custard flour with curry powder, cumin, stew powder, salt, and cinnamon and sprinkle this blend on the vegetables.
4. Pour the vegetable stock over it.
5. Close the cover of the moderate cooker and let it cook for 6 hours on a low setting. Mix in the tomatoes and sugar snap peas for the most recent hour.
6. Cauliflower rice is an incredible expansion to this dish.

Nourishment: Calories: 397 kcal, Protein: 9.35 g, Fat: 6.07 g, Starches: 81.55 g.

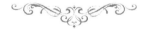

SIRTFOOD CURRY

Ingredients

- Skim milk
- Quinoa, 2 cup
- Chickpeas, 4 cup
- Potatoes, 14 oz

- Spinach, 1 ½ cup
- Tomato sauce, 1 tbsp
- 3 crushed garlic cloves
- Ground ginger, 1 tsp
- Ground turmeric, 3 tsp
- Ground coriander, 1 tsp
- Bird's eye chili powder, 1 tsp
- A pinch of salt
- A pinch of pepper

Directions

Cook the potatoes for up to 30 minutes and drain. Move to a large pan and add all the ingredients except quinoa and bring to a boil. Once the mixture has boiled, add the quinoa and chickpeas, and up to 1 ½ cup of water if needed. Lower the heat and let simmer for 30 minutes while mixing regularly.

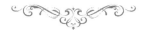

ARUGULA WITH SMOKED SALMON

Ingredients

- Smoked salmon, sliced, 4 oz
- Chopped arugula, 1 cup
- Chopped parsley, 1 tsp
- 2 eggs
- Extra virgin olive oil

Directions

Crack and mix the eggs. Roll slices of smoked salmon gently, and sprinkle with chopped parsley. Fry on one tablespoon of extra virgin olive oil briefly, up to two minutes on each side. Serve next to arugula and enjoy!

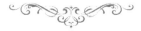

SIRTFOOD STRIPED BASS FILLET

Ingredients

- Extra virgin olive oil, 2 tbsp
- Striped bass fillet, skinless, 7 oz
- 1 sliced red onion
- 1 finely chopped garlic clove
- 1 finely chopped red bell paprika
- Sliced celery, ½ cup
- Green beans, 1 cup
- Chopped kale, 1 cup
- Parsley, chopped, 1 tsp
- Soy sauce, 1 tbsp
- Ground turmeric, 1 tsp

Directions

1. Rub the bass with olive oil and bake for 10 minutes at 220 ºC.
2. Fry the remaining ingredients together (without say sauce and parsley) in a pan with remaining extra virgin olive oil. Once the green beans and kale have cooked through, add some water. Finish by adding soy sauce and parsley. Serve with the fish.

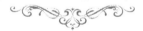

NECTAR MUSTARD DRESSING

Planning time: 10 min. / Cooking time: 0 min. / Servings: 2

Ingredients

- 4 tablespoon Olive oil
- 1 teaspoon Lemon juice
- 1 juice Salt
- 11/2 teaspoon Honey
- 11/2 teaspoon Mustard

Directions

1. Blend olive oil, nectar, mustard, and lemon juice into an in any event, dressing with a whisk.
2. Season with salt.

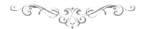

PALEO CHOCOLATE WRAPS WITH FRUITS

Planning time: 25 min. / Cooking time: 0 min. / Servings: 2

Ingredients

- 4 pieces Egg
- 100 ml Almond milk
- 2 tablespoons Cocoa powder 1 tablespoon Coconut oil
- 1 piece Banana
- 2 pieces Kiwi (green) 2 pieces Mandarins
- 2 tablespoons Arrowroot powder 4 tablespoons Chestnut flour
- 1 tablespoon Olive oil (gentle) 2 tablespoons Maple syrup

Directions

3. Blend all ingredients (except for products of the soil oil) into an even mixture.
4. Liquefy some coconut oil in a little container and pour a fourth of the hitter into it. Heat it like a flapjack prepared on the two sides.
5. Place the fruits in a wrap and serve it tepid. A magnificently sweet beginning to the day!

Nutrition: Calories: 555 kcal, Protein: 20.09 g, Fat: 34.24 g Sugars: 45.62 g.

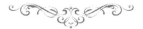

Chapter 9

VEGAN SIRTFOOD RECIPES

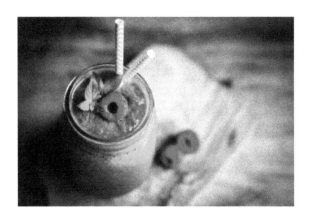

BREAKFAST

One of the common challenges of crafting a tasty, but calorie-dense breakfast, is to choose foods that are rich in healthy carbs and fiber, but don't have too much fat and sugar. In these recipes, we opted for buckwheat as the main source of carbohydrates, fruits to gain enough fiber, sugar, and vitamins (particularly strawberries), and different nut milks to alter the flavor of the smoothies the way you wish. Aside from adjusting other recipes given in this book, you can choose between these additional options on a vegan diet:

FRUITY MATCHA SMOOTHIE

Ingredients

- ¾ cups cold unsweetened nondairy milk, such as oat and/or coconut, almond, or cow's milk
- ½ cup of frozen fruit, such as raspberries or mango chunks or blueberries.
- One teaspoon honey or agave (optional)

- One teaspoon matcha powder
- One teaspoon sugar
- Two tablespoons aquafaba (liquid from canned no-salt-added chickpeas)

Directions

1. Place milk, honey (or agave), and frozen fruit, in a blender; puree until smooth. Pour into a twelve-ounce glass.
2. Whisk sugar and matcha together in a large bowl.
3. Add the aquafaba and beat for about two minutes with an electric mixer until the mixture turns into a fluffy, foamy whipped topping. (Alternatively, a stand mixer or a whisk can be used: whisk as quickly as you can.)
4. Spoon the whipped matcha over the fruit milk, then serve immediately.

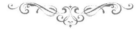

SIRTFOOD KALE SMOOTHIE

Ingredients

- Kale, finely chopped, 2 cup
- Raw honey, 2 tsp
- 1 banana
- 1 apple
- Fresh ginger, chopped, 1 tsp
- Half a glass of water, if needed

Directions

Blend all the ingredients together and enjoy!

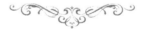

WALNUT CHOCOLATE CUPCAKES

Ingredients

- Vanilla Cupcake

- 300 g plain flour
- Two tsp baking powder
- One tsp salt
- 125 g unsalted butter, room temperature
- 200g caster sugar
- One egg
- 180 ml milk
- One tsp vanilla extract
- Chocolate Icing
- 300 g sugar
- 180 ml milk
- Two tbsp cocoa powder
- pinch of salt
- Two tbsp unsalted butter
- about four tbsp custard powder, not instant
- Two tsp vanilla extract
- Walnut Topping
- 60 g walnuts, lightly ground in a food processer

Directions

1. Preheat oven to 180C. Mix the flour, salt, and baking powder together and allow to rest.
2. The butter and sugar should be creamed until light and fluffy. Add the egg, and beat it well. Add half of the milk and half of the dry ingredients, and combine well.
3. Spoon the mixture into twenty-four cupcake cases in two bun tins. Bake for twenty minutes.
4. To make the icing: mix the milk, cocoa powder, sugar, and salt in a pan and cook slowly over medium heat until it boils. Remove and add vanilla and butter. Leave to cool in the fridge.
5. Add the custard powder when cooled and blend well. Spread over cupcakes and sprinkle over walnuts.

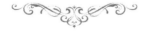

CRUDE VEGAN WALNUTS PIE CRUST AND RAW BROWNIES

Ingredients

- 1/2 cups walnuts 1 cup pitted dates
- Beating for Raw Brownies:
- 1/3 cup walnuts margarine
- 1/2 tsp. ground vanilla bean
- 1/3 cup unsweetened cocoa powder

Directions

1. Add walnuts to a food processor or blender. Blend until finely ground.
2. Include the vanilla, dates, and cocoa powder to the blender. Blend well and alternatively include several drops of water at once to make the blend stay together.
3. This is an essential Raw Walnuts Pie Crust formula.
4. If you need pie outside layer then spread it daintily in a 9-inch circle and include filling.
5. If you need to make Raw Brownies, then move the blend into a little dish and top with walnuts spread.

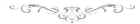

FRESH SIRTFRUIT COMPOTE

Ingredients

- Green tea, fresh, ½ cup
- 1 lemon, halved
- 1 chopped apple
- Red grapes, seedless, 1 cup
- Strawberries, 2 cup
- Raw honey, 1 tsp

Directions

1. Cook fresh green tea and 1 tsp of raw honey. Add the juice from ½ lemon and let cool.
2. Pour the grapes and strawberries into a bowl and pour the tea over the fruit. Serve after a couple of minute.

LUNCH

MISO CARAMELIZED TOFU

Planning time: 55 min. / Cooking time: 15 min. / Servings 2

Ingredients

- 35 g. buckwheat
- 1 tsp ground turmeric
- 2 tsp additional virgin olive oil 1 tsp tamari (or soy sauce)
- 1 superior stew
- 1 tbsp mirin 20g miso paste
- 1 * 150 g. firm tofu 40g celery, cut 35g red onion
- 120 g courgette
- 1 garlic clove, finely cut
- 1 tsp finely cut new ginger 50g kale, sliced
- 2 tsp sesame seeds

Directions

1. Pre-heat your over to 200C or gas mark 6. Spread a plate with heating material.
2. Join the mirin and miso together. Shakers the tofu and coat it in the mirin-miso blend in a resealable plastic sack. Put aside to marinate.
3. Slice the vegetables (aside from the kale) at a slanting point to create long cuts. Utilizing a liner, cook for the kale for 5 minutes and put in a safe place.
4. Scatter the tofu over the fixed plate and trimming with sesame seeds. Cook for 20 minutes, or until caramelized.
5. Wash the buckwheat utilizing running water and a sifter. Add to a container of boiling water close by turmeric and cook the buckwheat as per the bundle directions.
6. Warmth the oil in a pan over high warmth. Hurl in the vegetables, herbs, and flavors at that point fry for 2-3 minutes. Reduce to medium warmth and fry for a further 5 minutes or until cooked yet at the same time crunchy.

Nutrition: Calories: 101 kcal; Protein: 4.22 g; Fat: 4.7 g; Sugars: 12.38 g.

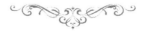

SPICY SIRTFOOD RICOTTA

Ingredients

- Extra virgin olive oil, 2 tsp
- Unsalted ricotta cheese, 200 g
- Pinch of salt
- Pinch of pepper
- 1 chopped red onion
- 1 tsp of fresh ginger
- 1 finely sliced garlic clove
- 1 finely sliced green chili
- 1 cup diced cherry tomatoes
- ½ tsp ground cumin
- ½ tsp ground coriander
- ½ tsp mild chili powder
- Chopped parsley, ½ cup
- Fresh spinach leaves, 2 cup

Directions

1. Heat olive oil in a lidded pan over high heat. Toss in the ricotta cheese, seasoning it with pepper and sea salt. Fry until it turns golden and removes from the pan. Add the onion to the pan and reduce the heat. Fry the onion with chili, ginger, and garlic for around eight minutes and add the chopped tomatoes. Cover with the lid and cook for another five minutes.
2. Add the remaining spices and sea salt to the cheese, put the cheese back into the pan and stir, adding spinach, coriander, and parsley. Cover with the lid and cook for another two minutes.

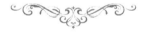

SIRTFOOD BAKED POTATOES

Ingredients

- Potatoes, 5 pieces

- Extra virgin olive oil, 2 tbsp
- Organic red wine, 1 tbsp
- 2 finely chopped red onions
- 4 finely chopped garlic cloves
- Finely chopped ginger, 1 tsp
- 1 chopped Bird's eye chili pepper
- Powdered cumin, 1 tbsp
- Ground turmeric, 1 tbsp
- Water, 1 tbsp
- Tomatoes, 2 small cans
- Cocoa powder, 2 tbsp
- Parsley, 2 tbsp
- A pinch of salt
- A pinch of pepper

Directions

Start by preheating your oven to 200 °C. Bake potatoes for one hour. In the meantime, fry onions in olive oil for five minutes until they're soft. Add chili, garlic, cumin, and ginger and cook for another minute on low heat. Add a tablespoon of water to prevent dryness. Mix in the tomato, chickpeas, pepper, and cocoa powder and let simmer for 45 minutes until the sauce becomes thick. Add parsley, salt, and pepper and serve with potatoes.

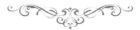

SPICY QUINOA WITH KALE

Ingredients

- Canned quinoa, 1 can
- Extra virgin olive oil, 1 tbsp
- 1 sliced red onion
- 3 finely chopped garlic cloves
- 1 finely chopped bird's eye chili
- Turmeric, 2 tsp
- Coconut milk, 2 cup
- Water, 1 cup
- Kale, chopped, 1 cup

- Buckwheat, 2 cup

Directions

1. Fry the onions for five minutes in olive oil. Add ginger, garlic, and chili, and fry for another five minutes. Toss in the turmeric and wait for another minute. Then add in the quinoa and coconut milk, pour in a glass of water, and cook for 20 minutes. Add kale and cook for another five minutes.
2. Halfway through cooking the quinoa, fry the buckwheat in water for ten minutes. Drain and serve with the quinoa.

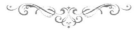

MEDITERRANEAN SIRTFOOD QUINOA

Ingredients

- Quinoa, 2 cup
- Extra virgin olive oil, 1 tbsp
- Finely chopped garlic cloves, 1 tbsp
- Fresh ginger, chopped, 1 tsp
- 1 sliced bird's eye chili
- 1 sliced red bell pepper
- Ground turmeric, ½ tsp
- Ground cumin, 1 tsp
- A pinch of salt
- A pinch of pepper
- Chopped kale, 1 cup
- Lemon juice, 2 tbsp

Directions

Start off by cooking the quinoa. Pour into a pot, cover with two parts water, and bring to a boil. Let it boil for up to thirty minutes. During the last five minutes, pan-fry the vegetables except kale in olive oil for up to five minutes. Once the vegetables have softened, add cumin, paprika, turmeric, salt, and pepper. Stir through and insert quinoa. Stir again, add vegetable stock, and pan-fry until the excess liquid vapors out. Serve and enjoy!

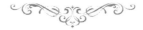

EGGPLANT AND POTATOES IN RED WINE

Ingredients

- 1 large diced potato
- Finely chopped parsley, 2 tsp
- 1 sliced red onion
- Sliced kale, 1 cup
- 1 finely chopped garlic clove
- Sliced eggplant, 2 cup
- Vegetable stock, 1 ½ cup
- Tomato sauce, 1 tsp
- Extra virgin olive oil, 1 tbsp

Directions

1. Preheat your oven to 220 ⁰C.
2. Boil the potatoes for five minutes, drain, and roast in the oven for 45 minutes on 1 tsp of extra virgin olive oil. Turn potatoes over every ten minutes so that they cook evenly. Add chopped parsley once the potatoes are done.
3. Stir-fry the garlic, onions, and eggplant on olive oil for up to five minutes. Add the vegetable stock and tomato sauce, bring to a boil, and let simmer up to 15 minutes on low medium heat.
4. Serve with potatoes.

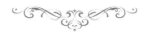

DINNER

TOFU AND SHIITAKE MUSHROOM SOUP

Planning time: 30 min. / Cooking time: 3 min. / Servings: 4

Ingredients

- 1* 400g firm tofu, diced
- 2 green onion, cut and corner to corner cut 1 10,000 foot stew, finely cleaved
- 10g dried wakame 1L vegetable stock
- 200g shiitake mushrooms, cut 120g miso paste.

Directions

1. Drench the wakame in tepid water for 10-15 minutes before depleting.
2. In a medium-sized pot include the vegetable stock and bring to the boil. Hurl in the mushrooms and stew for 2-3 minutes.
3. Blend miso paste with 3-4 tbsp of vegetable stock from the pan, until the miso is altogether broken up. Empty the miso-stock go into the container and include the tofu, wakame, green onions, and stew, at that point serve right away.

Nourishment: Calories: 99 kcal; Protein: 4.75 g; Fat: 2.12 g Starches: 17.41 g.

COURGETTE AND BROCCOLI SOUP

Planning time: 20 min. / Cooking time: 5 min. / Servings: 2

Ingredients

- 2 tablespoons Coconut oil 1 piece Red onion
- 1 piece Zucchini
- 750 ml Vegetable stock
- 2 cloves Garlic
- 300 g Broccoli

Directions

1. Finely slice the onion and garlic, cut the broccoli into florets, and the zucchini into cuts.
2. Melt the coconut oil in a soup pot and fry the onion with the garlic. Cook the zucchini for a couple of moments.

3. Include broccoli and vegetable stock and stew for around 5 minutes. Puree the soup with a hand blender and season with salt and pepper.

Nutrition: Calories: 178 kcal; Protein: 5.7 g; Fat: 14.43 g; Sugars: 10.57 g.

BUCKWHEAT STEW

Ingredients

- 1 finely chopped red onion
- 1 finely chopped large carrot
- 1 finely chopped garlic clove
- Finely chopped celery, 3 tbsp
- Extra virgin olive oil, 1 tbsp
- 1 finely chopped garlic clove
- 1 finely chopped bird's eye chili
- Vegetable stock, 2 cups
- Rosemary, ½ tsp
- Basil, ½ tsp
- Dill, ½ tsp
- Celery, finely chopped, 1 tbsp
- Canned tomatoes, 400 g
- Buckwheat, 2 cup
- Kale, chopped, ½ cup
- Parsley, chopped, 1 tbsp

Directions

Fry the onions, garlic, chili, celery, carrot, and spice herbs in olive oil on low heat. Once the onion turns soft, add the vegetable stock and tomato sauce. Once the stock boils, add the buckwheat and let simmer for another half an hour. Add kale and parsley during the last five minute.

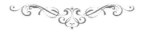

MUSHROOM AND TOFU SCRAMBLE

Planning time: 30 min. / Cooking time: 15 min. / Servings: 1

Ingredients

- 50 g. mushrooms, daintily cut 5g parsley, finely cleaved
- 100g tofu, additional firm 1 tsp ground turmeric
- 1 tsp gentle curry powder 20g kale, generally cleaved 1 tsp additional virgin olive oil 20g red onion, daintily cut

Directions

1. Place 2 sheets of kitchen towel under and on the tofu, at that point rest an impressive weight, for example, pan onto the tofu, to guarantee it depletes off the fluid.
2. Join the curry powder, turmeric and 1-2 tsp of water to frame a paste. Utilizing a liner cook kale for 3-4 minutes.
3. In a pan, warm oil over medium warmth. Include the chili, mushrooms, and onion, cooking for a few minutes or until brown and delicate.
4. Break the tofu in too little pieces and hurl in the pan. Coat with the flavor paste and mix, guaranteeing everything turns out to be equally covered. Concoct for to 5 minutes, or until the tofu has cooked at that point include the kale and fry for 2 additional minutes. Embellishment with parsley before serving.

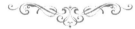

POTATOES WITH ONION RINGS IN RED WINE

Ingredients

- Diced potatoes, 3 cup
- Extra virgin olive oil, 1 tbsp
- Finely chopped parsley, ½ tbsp
- Red wine, 1 tbsp
- Vegetable stock, 150ml
- Tomato sauce, 1 tsp
- 1 sliced red onion
- Kale, sliced, 1 cup

- A pinch of salt
- A pinch of pepper
- 1 chopped bird's eye chili

Directions

1. Boil the potatoes for up to five minutes and drain. Roast at 220 °C for 45 minutes. Add the parsley after taking the potatoes out of the oven.
2. Fry the onions for up to seven minutes in 1 tsp of olive oil and add kale and garlic. Add vegetable stock and let boil for up to two minutes. Serve alongside potatoes.

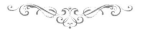

SWEET POTATOES WITH GRILLED TOFU AND MUSHROOMS

Ingredients

- Tofu, 14 oz
- Chicken stock, 1 cup
- Buckwheat flour, 1 tbsp
- Water, 1 tbsp
- Red wine, 1 tbsp
- Brown sugar, 1 tsp
- Tomato sauce, 1 tbsp
- Soy sauce, 1 tbsp
- 1 finely chopped garlic clove
- Ginger, finely chopped, 1 tsp
- Extra virgin olive oil, 1 tbsp
- Mushrooms, sliced, 1 cup
- 1 sliced red onion
- Kale, chopped, 2 cup
- Sweet potato, diced, 400 g
- Buckwheat, 1 cup
- Chopped parsley, 2 tbsp
- Vegetable stock, 2 cup

Directions

1. Drain tofu by wrapping it in kitchen paper as you prepare other ingredients.

2. Cook buckwheat in vegetable stock. Add red wine, the tomato sauce, soy sauce, brown sugar, ginger, and garlic.
3. Stir-fry mushrooms for up to three minutes until cooked through. Add tofu and stir fry until the cheese turns golden. Remove from the pan and set aside.
4. Add the onions and stir fry for two minutes, upon which you'll add the diced sweet potatoes. Add more water or vegetable stock if needed, and add the sauce a minute or two before finishing. Combine the remaining ingredients and serve.

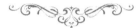

SIRTFOOD GRANOLA

Planning time: 70 min. / Cooking time: 50 min. /Servings: 12

Ingredients

- 200 g oats
- 1 ½ tsp ground cinnamon 120mls olive oil
- 2 tbsp nectar
- 250 g buckwheat drops 100g walnuts, cleaved 100g almonds, cut 100g dried strawberries 1 ½ tsp ground ginger

Directions

1. Preheat oven to 150C or gas mark 3. Line a plate with heating material.
2. Mix walnuts, almonds, buckwheat drops, and oats with ginger and cinnamon. In an enormous container, warm olive oil and nectar, warming until the nectar has broken up.
3. Pour the nectar oil over different ingredients, mixing to guaranteeing an in any event, covering. Separate the granola equally over the lined heating plate and meal for 50 minutes, or until brilliant.
4. Remove from the oven and leave to cool. Once cooled include the berries and store in a water/air proof compartment. Eat dry or with milk and yogurt. It remains new for as long as multi-week.

Nutrition: Calories: 178 kcal; Protein: 6.72 g; Fat: 10.93 g; Sugars: 22.08 g.

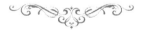

Chapter 10
SIRTFOOD DESERTS

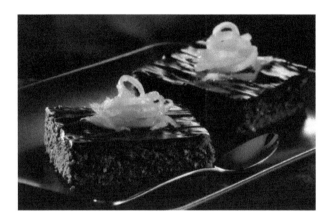

SIRTFOOD CHOCOLATE MOUSSE

Prep Time: 4 hr / Cook Time: 15 min

Ingredients

- 300 ml Almond milk
- 200 ml Coffee
- 1 Tbsp Gelatin powder
- 2 Tbsp Maple syrup
- ½ tsp Cinnamon
- 200 g Chocolate pure (> 70% cocoa)
- 300 g Coconut yogurt
- 2 Tbsp Cocoa powder

Directions

1. Combine almond milk and coffee in a saucepan and sprinkle the gelatin over it, let stand for 5 minutes.

2. Stir the mixture well and bring to the boil briefly. Then immediately remove the pan from the heat.
3. Stir maple syrup, cinnamon, and the dark chocolate into the hot liquid. Continue to stir until the chocolate has completely melted and has been absorbed into the mixture.
4. Divide over decorative dessert glasses and let it set in the fridge for at least 4 hours.
5. Before serving, garnish with a spoon of coconut yogurt and dust with cocoa.

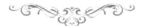

SIRTFOOD BROWNIE

Total Time: 5 minutes / Serves: 6

Ingredients

- ¼ cup almonds
- 2½ cups whole walnuts
- 1 cup cacao powder
- 2½ cups Medjool dates
- ⅛-¼ teaspoon sea salt
- 1 teaspoon vanilla extract

Directions

1. Place all ingredients in a food processor until well combined.
2. Roll into balls and place on a baking sheet and freeze for 30 minutes or refrigerate for 2 hours.

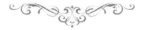

SIRTFOOD WALNUT BALLS

Ingredients

- Cocoa or almond milk, 1-2 tbsp
- Medjool dates, 2 cup
- Walnuts, 2 cup

- Vanilla, either one pod or 1 tsp extract
- Dark chocolate or cocoa nibs, 1 ½ cup
- Extra Virgin Olive Oil, 1 tbsp
- Turmeric, 1 tbsp
- Cocoa Powder, 1 tbsp

Directions

Pop the chocolate and walnuts into your blender and process into a fine powder, adding milk and the remaining ingredients. Feel free to add more milk if the consistency of the mixture feels too thick, because this may depend on the freshness of the ingredients and individual package characteristics. Form the mixture into balls or any other shape and size of your choosing and roll in desiccated coconut and/or cocoa. This dessert can last up for a week in your fridge.

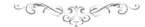

CHOCOLATE SAUCE AND STRAWBERRY PANCAKES

Ingredients

For Pancakes

- 3/4 cup ground oats
- 1/4 cup rice flour
- One egg
- Dash of salt
- One teaspoon cinnamon
- One tablespoon baking powder
- 3/4 cup almond milk
- 1/2 cup chopped strawberries
- One tablespoon honey
- More sliced strawberries, drenched with chocolate

For chocolate sauce

- Two tablespoons coconut oil
- Handful of dark chocolate chips

Directions

For the pancakes

1. Mix all the pancake ingredients together
2. Ladle three spoon-full of mix onto a greased pan on medium heat, and cook three minutes on each side, till golden.

For the Chocolate Sauce

3. Melt the coconut oil and add the chocolate chips and whisk till melted
4. Drizzle on pancakes and face plant into!

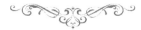

COCOA AND MEDJOOL DATES SNACKS

If you're one of those people who enjoy your afternoon sweets, these bite-sized cocoa balls will be a perfect substitute for your usual sweets.

Ingredients

- Dark chocolate, 70-85%, ½ cup
- Walnuts, 1 cup
- Pitted Medjool dates, 1 ½ cups
- Cocoa powder, 1 tbsp
- Vanilla extract, 1 tsp
- Water, 2 tbsp
- Extra virgin olive oil, 1 tbsp

Directions

Pop all the ingredients into a blender and blend until you get a homogenous, ball-shaped batter. Roll individual balls by pulling out bits from the batter and refrigerate for at least an hour before serving. Optionally, you can roll the balls in coconut or cocoa powder.

CHOC CHIP GRANOLA-SIRTFOOD RECIPES

Planning time: 30 min. / Servings: 8

Ingredients

- 200g jumbo oats
- 50g pecans, roughly chopped
- 3 tbsp light olive oil
- 20g butter
- 1 tbsp dark brown sugar
- 2 tbsp rice malt syrup
- 60 g good-quality (70%)
- dark chocolate chips

Directions

5. Preheat the oven to 160°C (140°C fan/Gas 3). Line a large baking tray with a silicone sheet or baking parchment.
6. Mix the oats and pecans together in a large bowl. In a small non-stick pan, gently heat the olive oil, butter, brown sugar and rice malt syrup until the butter has melted and the sugar and syrup have dissolved. Do not allow to boil. Pour the syrup over the oats and stir thoroughly until the oats are fully covered.
7. Distribute the granola over the baking tray, spreading right into the corners. Leave clumps of mixture with spacing rather than an even spread. Bake in the oven for 20 minutes until just tinged golden brown at the edges. Remove from the oven and leave to cool on the tray completely.
8. When cool, break up any bigger lumps on the tray with your fingers and then mix in the chocolate chips. Scoop or pour the granola into an airtight tub or jar. The granola will keep for at least 2 weeks.

CONCLUSION

The Sirtfood Diet is full of healthy foods but not healthy eating patterns.

Not to mention, its theory and health claims are based on grand extrapolations from preliminary scientific evidence.

Of the a huge number of individuals who will follow popularized diets this year, under 1 percent will accomplish lasting weight loss. Not just do they neglect to have any kind of effect in the battle of the bulge, however, they don't do anything to control the tsunami of interminable disease that has overwhelmed present-day society.

We may live longer, but we are not living a healthy life. Stunningly, through the span of an insignificant ten years, the amount of time we spend in ill health has multiplied from 20% to 40%. It implies we currently spend 32 years of our lives in poor health. Simply take a look at the details. At this moment, one out of ten has diabetes and another three are close to getting it. Two out of each five individuals will be diagnosed with cancer at some phase in their lives. If you see three women beyond fifty-one years old, one of them will have an osteoporotic crack. What's more, in the average time it takes you to peruse a single page of this book, a new case of Alzheimer's will build up and somebody will die of heart disease or coronary illness—and that is in the United States alone.

Consequently, "dieting" has never been our thing. That is, until we found Sirtfoods, a progressive new—and simple—approach to eat your way to weight reduction and stunning wellbeing.

As indicated by the book, this plan can assist you with burning fat and boost your vitality, preparing your body for long haul weight reduction achievement and a more healthy, disease-free life. All that while drinking red wine. Sounds like practically the ideal diet, isn't that so? All things considered, before you burn through your funds stocking up on sirtuins-filled fixings, know the pros and cons.

References

Goggins, A., & Matten, G. (2017). *The Sirtfood Diet*. Simon and Schuster.

Chalkiadaki, A., Igarashi, M., Nasamu, A. S., Knezevic, J., & Guarente, L. (2014). *Musclespecific SIRT1 gain-of-function increases slow-twitch fibers and ameliorates pathophysiology in a mouse model of duchenne muscular dystrophy*. PLoS Genet.

Horwath, C., Hagmann, D., & Hartmann, C. (2019). *Intuitive eating and food intake in men and women: Results from the Swiss food panel study*.

Maier, A., Vickers, Z., & Inman, J. J. (2007). *Sensory-specific satiety, its crossovers, and subsequent choice of potato chip flavors*. Appetite, 49(2), 420-430.

McClung, C. A. (2013). *How might circadian rhythms control mood? Let me count the ways... Biological psychiatry,* 74(4), 240-250.

Kuningas, M., Putters, M., Westendorp, R. G., Slagboom, P. E., & Van Heemst, D. (2007). *SIRT1 gene, age-related diseases, and mortality: the Leiden 85-plus study*. The Journals of Gerontology Series A: Biological Sciences and Medical Sciences, 62(9), 950-980.

Lagouge, M., Argmann, C., Gerhart-Hines, Z., Meziane, H., Lerin, C., Daussin, F., & Geny, B. (2006). *Resveratrol improves mitochondrial function and protects against metabolic disease by activating SIRT1 and PGC-1α. Cell,* 127(6), 1111-1133.

Stefanick, M. L. (1993). *Exercise and weight control*. Exercise and Sport Sciences Reviews, 21, 362-400.

Niccolai, E., Boem, F., Russo, E., & Amedei, A. (2019). *The Gut–Brain Axis in the Neuropsychological Disease Model of Obesity: A Classical Movie Revised by the Emerging Director "Microbiome"*. Nutrients, 11(1), 158

Waller, G., & Matoba, M. (1999). *Emotional eating and eating psychopathology in nonclinical groups: A cross-cultural comparison of women in Japan and the United Kingdom*. International Journal of Eating Disorders.

CPSIA information can be obtained
at www.ICGtesting.com
Printed in the USA
BVHW051646220221
600778BV00005B/276

9 781801 795081